Barbi
Sil

# control
# IBS
## irritable bowel syndrome

## your
# 7-day
# diet
# plan

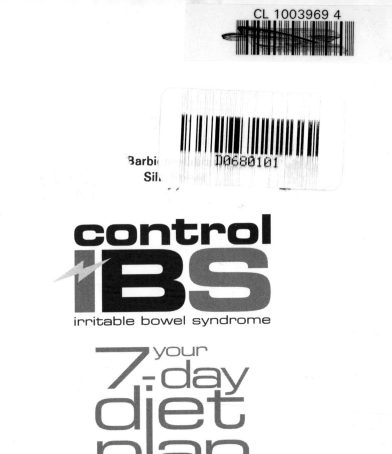

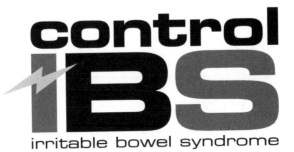

# control IBS

## irritable bowel syndrome

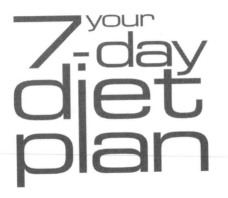

your 7-day diet plan

## carolyn humphries

foulsham

LONDON • NEW YORK • TORONTO • SYDNEY

# foulsham

The Publishing House, Bennetts Close, Cippenham,
Slough, Berkshire, SL1 5AP, England

Foulsham books can be found in all good bookshops and direct
from www.foulsham.com

ISBN-13: 978-0-572-03228-9
ISBN-10: 0-572-03228-5

Cover photograph © Terry Pastor

A CIP record for this book is available from the British Library

The moral right of the author has been asserted

Neither the editors of W. Foulsham & Co. Ltd nor the
author nor the publisher take responsibility for any
possible consequences from any treatment, procedure,
test, exercise, action or application of medication or
preparation by any person reading or following the
information in this book. The publication of this book
does not constitute the practice of medicine, and this
book does not attempt to replace any diet or
instructions from your doctor. The author and
publisher advise the reader to check with a doctor
before administering any medication or undertaking
any course of treatment or exercise.

Printed in Great Britain by Creative Print and Design (Wales), Ebbw Vale

# CONTENTS

# INTRODUCTION

Irritable bowel syndrome (IBS) is a very common condition that makes the intestines oversensitive, leading to a variety of abdominal and bowel symptoms. As many as one in five people suffers from IBS in varying degrees. There is no cure but it can be managed with a healthy lifestyle, including regular exercise and a diet rich in foods that can ease the symptoms and that avoids the trigger foods.

This book tells you all you need to know about the condition, how to cope with it and when to seek medical advice. It also provides a complete eating plan, including a repertoire of fabulous, tasty, easy-to-prepare meals for every occasion.

# WHAT IS IBS?

Irritable bowel syndrome is very common and affects millions of people worldwide – almost as many working days are lost because of IBS as for the common cold! It can affect people at any age but usually appears at some time from the teens onwards.

Despite being so widespread, it is commonly misunderstood – perhaps largely because it is a topic most people prefer to keep private. In fact, it is often called the 'misunderstood disease' because so many people believe it is a psychological condition rather than a real illness. This is not so. Although psychological influences can instigate or exacerbate an attack, the effect on the bowel is very real indeed – as sufferers know only too well.

The exact cause of IBS has not been identified, but it is known that the symptoms are caused by a loss of co-ordination between the two types of muscular contractions that cause food to move through the gut (something you are not aware of when everything is functioning normally). The disorder can affect the whole digestive tract, or sometimes only one part – so you might just feel a lump in the throat and food getting stuck there if that's the area that's affected, or experience diarrhoea and/or constipation if the problem occurs further down.

IBS should not be confused with ulcerative colitis or Crohn's disease, both of which cause serious inflammation of the colon.

## SYMPTOMS OF IBS

IBS causes a variety of symptoms. If you experience any one of those listed below, there may well be another cause, but if you suffer several of them on a regular basis you should see your doctor for a diagnosis.

- A feeling that your throat is constricted between meals, but you are still able to swallow.

- Heartburn.

- Rapidly feeling full when eating a meal, so you can't finish your portion.

- Loud, frequent gurgling in the stomach (not just the odd little one, which is normal).

- Bloating.

- Large amounts of flatulence.

- Excessive burping.

- Bad breath.

- Frequent stomach pains.

- Abdominal cramps that don't go away when the bowels have been opened.

- A tender abdomen.

- Diarrhoea.

- Constipation.

- Bouts of constipation followed by bouts of diarrhoea (this is different from a one-off situation of not going to the loo for a couple of days after having had a bout of diarrhoea, which is quite normal).

- The inability to control the bowels properly – the sensation of having to rush to the loo with clenched cheeks.

- Inability to open the bowels easily and feeling that they are not emptied fully.

- Short sharp stabbing pains in the rectum.

- Nausea.

- Frequent tiredness.

- Unexplained headaches.

## SYMPTOMS THAT SHOULD NOT
## BE ASCRIBED TO IBS

Any of the following symptoms must be checked out by your doctor because they could be caused by something more serious than IBS that needs expert medical attention.

- A bloated stomach that doesn't ease overnight.

- Indigestion-like pain in the night.

- A problem with swallowing so food gets stuck in your throat.

- Rapid weight loss for no reason.

- Persistent watery diarrhoea.

- Bleeding from the back passage.

- Blood in your stools.

- Mucus in your stools.

## WHAT BRINGS ON AN ATTACK?

The bowels are very sensitive; even people who don't suffer from the syndrome may well get an attack of diarrhoea when they are anxious, such as going for a job interview or to the dentist. Certain foods and drinks are known to aggravate the problem (see pages 16–17) but you may also find that stress plays a large part.

If you suffer from several of the symptoms on pages 8–9 on a regular basis, I recommend you see your doctor. You should be given an abdominal examination and have blood taken for testing, and should also be offered medical procedures such as x-rays to exclude other major problems. If your symptoms are severe – including bleeding from the back passage, loss of appetite and noticeable weight loss – or there is a history of breast, stomach, bowel, ovarian or womb cancer in your family you may be referred to a specialist who is likely to give you a more detailed examination of your abdomen, an examination of the back passage and, possibly, a barium enema and/or a colonoscopy (an internal examination of your colon with a very fine camera). Quite often, after all that, your doctor will say there is nothing visibly wrong. It will depend on the physician what treatment you are offered as some are more sympathetic than others. But don't despair because the following chapters on diet and lifestyle will help no end.

# COMMON TREATMENTS FOR IBS

If nothing untoward is found by your doctor or from hospital investigations, it is very likely that your condition is IBS. There is a variety of treatments available and it will depend on your doctor what you are offered.

## POSSIBLE TREATMENT OPTIONS

These may include any of the following options.

- Concentrated peppermint oil capsules.

- Drugs that ease bowel spasms may help to stop the pain you are experiencing. They either work by affecting the muscle in the bowel wall itself or by convincing the nervous system that it is calm, so the bowel doesn't react.

- A proprietary product such as Imodium®, which stops diarrhoea by slowing the rate of bowel contractions.

- Laxatives if constipated (though these can do more harm than good if taken regularly).

- In severe cases, a low-dosage antidepressant may be given to calm the nervous system and thus stop the bowel movements.

- Fibre supplements.

- Antacid medicine.

If you prefer, you might like to explore homeopathic remedies. One of the following could help but I would urge you to talk to a homeopath before taking any of them, as he or she will take a holistic approach and so treat your whole body, not just the specific problem.

- **Argentum nitricum** This may be suggested if your symptoms are brought on by stress and anxiety, particularly if they include diarrhoea, nausea, flatulence and bloating.

- **Asafoetida** This can help if you feel that your throat is constricted, you are bloated but are unable to relieve it by belching or breaking wind, you are slightly sick after eating or have stomach pains and constipation or acute diarrhoea.

- **Colocynthis** This is said to be good if you have cramps in your lower abdomen and diarrhoea.

- **Lilium tigrinum** This is recommended to treat bouts of constipation followed by diarrhoea or a feeling that the bowels don't empty fully and that a lump of stool remains.

- **Lycopodium** This may be helpful if you often start to feel full early on when eating a meal or suffer from bloating, heartburn, flatulence and stomach pain.

- **Natrum carbonicum** If you are sure your IBS is associated with food intolerances, such as lactose or wheat/gluten, then this may be suggested.

- **Nux vomica** If you are stressed and have constipation, abdominal pain or cramps and flatulence, this is a possible solution.

# HOW TO HELP YOURSELF

As with any condition, IBS will be affected by what you do, so it makes sense to try to minimise the situations that aggravate the condition and do everything you can to alleviate it, or stop if flaring up in the first place.

## PREVENTION IS BETTER THAN CURE

This may be a cliché, but it is true! The first step is to try to prevent attacks and there are many things you can do to help.

First and foremost, try to stop feeling so anxious about it. The condition is manageable but worrying will just make things worse!

- Eat a healthy, well-balanced diet (see pages 18–21) including plenty of fresh fruit and vegetables, and soluble and insoluble fibre. If you have constipation, increase your fibre intake immediately by eating lots of whole grains, nuts, seeds, dried fruit etc. If you suffer from diarrhoea, you still need to increase fibre but take it a little more gradually, introducing one new high-fibre food at a time.

- Always eat starchy foods at the start of the meal to 'line' the stomach, especially at breakfast.

- Always eat insoluble fibre (the husk on grains and tough fibres on vegetables and fruit) with other foods. Don't add extra wheat bran to your food.

- Eat raw fruit or vegetables (such as salad) at the end of the meal, not at the beginning. Always cut it up well and chew it thoroughly. If raw foods seem to cause problems, cook them lightly first.

- Always skin and seed food with pips, such as tomatoes, cucumber and (bell) peppers. It makes them much easier to digest.

- Identify and avoid any trigger foods (see pages 16–17). The best way to do this is to keep a food diary of everything you eat on a daily basis. Then, when you get an attack, you may well be able to work out which foods caused the problem. Then try eliminating them from your diet and see if this helps.

- Don't eat your main meal late at night. Either have it at lunch time or in the early evening.
- Avoid rich and fatty foods.
- Don't fry foods. Grilled (broiled), steamed or poached is much better for you.
- Don't have take-aways or ready meals very often; they will make your condition worse.
- Eat small meals on a regular basis rather than one or two large blow-outs a day. I recommend three meals with two nutritious snacks in between.
- Drink plenty of water every day – preferably six to eight glasses!
- Take exercise regularly, both energetic and gentle.
- Try to avoid stressful situations.
- Learn to relax (see pages 22–24) and to sleep well and soundly (see pages 24–25).
- If you smoke – give it up!

## FOODS THAT CAN HELP

These foods can often help IBS symptoms and will contribute to a healthy, balanced diet.

- Buttermilk.
- Dried fruit (especially if you are constipated, but introduce it gradually if you have diarrhoea).
- Eggs (if egg yolks are a trigger food, use whites only).
- Fish.
- Fresh fruit and vegetables, peeled, cut up small or cooked.
- Ginger.
- Linseed.
- Live bio yoghurt.

- Nuts (preferably ground or chopped small) and seeds.
- Olive and sunflower oil.
- Peppermint.
- Skinless white meat (chicken, turkey, duck, game birds and rabbit).
- Starchy foods like pasta, rice and bread.
- Water – six to eight glasses a day.
- Whole grains, especially oats, barley and rye.

## FOODS THAT MAY IRRITATE

These are the most common foods that IBS sufferers have identified as culprits. But they won't all affect you – and you may find that there are others not listed here that cause your problems. I must emphasise that it is unwise to cut out whole ranges of foods on a whim. Keep your food diary and try to identify which individual foods cause problems, then eliminate them from your diet. Always make sure you are still maintaining a healthy balance (see pages 18–21). Don't avoid foods just because they are on the list – only do so if you are sure they cause or aggravate your own symptoms.

- Acidic fruits – citrus, tomatoes (may be tolerated if seeded and chopped first). If you must avoid them, try soft fruits instead, but always peeled, cored, stoned (pitted) and chopped or sliced. A tiny dash of lemon juice or a small squeeze of tomato purée in a dish may be fine even if you can't tolerate whole fruit. Trial and error is the key to finding your tolerance levels.
- Alcohol (it is usually fine when used in cooking).
- Bran – that is extra bran, added to your food.
- Caffeine in coffee, tea and cola – choose caffeine-free varieties.
- Chocolate – cocoa (unsweetened chocolate) powder should be fine, it's just the hard stuff that causes problems!

- Deep-fried foods and foods with a high fat content, so always choose low-fat dairy products, remove the skin from chicken and so on.

- Egg yolks (for omelettes, scrambled or for binding other foods, use whites only).

- Highly spiced foods – however, sweet spices such as cumin, cinnamon, mixed (apple pie) spice and Chinese five-spice actually aid digestion. Just avoid chilli and all its derivatives.

- Mayonnaise. Low-fat may be fine but, if not, use low-fat crème fraîche or buttermilk and flavour it with onion or garlic granules or a dash of Worcestershire sauce instead.

- Onions, leeks and garlic. Finely chopped and cooked well may be all right; if not, avoid and use onion or garlic granules for flavour or omit altogether.

- Pulses (dried peas, beans and lentils), which can cause flatulence (see the note for vegetarians on page 21 as pulses are very nutritious). Cooking them thoroughly and mashing or puréeing them will make them much more digestible.

- Red meat (beef, lamb, pork, venison); choose white meat like chicken, turkey, duck or rabbit instead.

- Sorbitol. This is an artificial sweetener often used in low-calorie foods, particularly sugar-free mints.

- Vinegar.

Cow's milk and some cheeses may cause problems, in which case you are probably lactose intolerant. Wheat and gluten (a protein found in wheat, barley, rye and oats) can also trigger IBS-like symptoms. However, do not exclude either of these food groups unless advised by your doctor to do so.

It is vital that you eat a balanced diet from the main food groups. Rather than dividing them into carbohydrates, proteins and so on, I have grouped them according to what you actually eat. You must have foods from all the groups below on a daily basis, in the proportions suggested. Whether you suffer from constipation or diarrhoea, it is important that you have plenty of natural fibre in your diet – particularly the soluble kind, which is found in most starchy foods. Insoluble fibre (the coarse husk on grains and fibrous tissue of vegetables) is also good for keeping the digestive system working, but when you have IBS you should always make sure you don't eat it on an empty stomach and don't have too much bran, so don't add it to your food. The amount of insoluble fibre that appears naturally in whole grains is absolutely fine.

I would also stress that, if you have previously had a low-fibre diet – for instance lots of processed white bread, white grains and little fruit and vegetables – you should introduce your new regime slowly and when you are free from an attack, particularly if you have diarrhoea regularly.

I would also suggest that, if your symptoms are severe and you find you are not eating enough fruit and vegetables, in particular, you take a multi-vitamin and mineral tablet daily.

## Cereals, grains and potatoes

These are starchy foods or fuel to give you the energy to do everything from sleeping and thinking to running a marathon. They will also fill you up, keep you warm and provide natural soluble and insoluble fibre. Half of what you eat every day should come from this group, which includes potatoes, yams, sweet potatoes, pasta, rice, oats and other grains, polenta, couscous, bulghar (cracked wheat), every type of bread and breakfast cereals.

Starchy foods are essential to health and, for the record, they won't make you fat (unless eaten in vast quantities) – it's the oodles of butter, other fats or sugary products you pile on them that do the damage. And you don't need to eat all wholegrain foods; a good mixture of white and brown is best for IBS sufferers.

## Fruit and vegetables

The more fruit and vegetables you eat the better for your health and well being. They provide essential vitamins, minerals and fibre and will help prevent heart disease and cancer. The group includes every type of fruit and vegetable you can lay your hands on – fresh, frozen, dried, canned (preferably in natural juice or water), nuts, seeds and pure fruit and vegetable juices. You should aim to eat at least five portions a day (a portion is a piece of fruit, a glass of juice or an average serving of vegetables).

Some people find that raw foods cause more problems than cooked. If this is the case, try shredding salad vegetables finely, which makes them easier to digest, or stick to cooked vegetables. Peeling fruit, cutting it up small and chewing it thoroughly will also help.

If cabbages and brassicas cause you flatulence, don't avoid them. They are so good for you so, instead, try cooking them slightly more than is normally recommended or finely chop or purée them and always use the cooking water in a sauce, gravy or soup so you don't lose all the nutrients.

Note that papayas (pawpaws) and mangos are particularly good for IBS sufferers as they aid digestion.

## Meat and other proteins

Proteins are vital for growth and repair of all body tissue. You'll find them in red meat such as lamb, pork and beef, poultry, fish, eggs (it's the white that contains the protein), and vegetable sources like dried peas, beans and lentils, soya protein, tofu and quorn.

There are some proteins – such as pork and beef – that have been known to make IBS worse in some people. If so, you may need to omit these from your diet and make sure you have alternative sources of protein. Beans and lentils are best served mashed or puréed to help prevent flatulence.

You don't need that much of this group, though, but it is important to eat a variety – 2–3 small portions a day is enough (about 10–15 per cent of your total food intake).

## Dairy products

Milk, cheese and yoghurt provide calcium for healthy teeth and bones. If you don't get enough, you risk osteoporosis (brittle bones) in later life as well as rotten teeth. However, you don't want too much fat so choose low-fat options where appropriate. Edam cheese is naturally lower in fat than other hard cheeses and is very versatile. If you can't tolerate dairy products, you can get enough of this group of nutrients from soya, oat, sunflower, nut or rice milks enriched with calcium, dried fruit, eggs, and dark green vegetables such as spinach and broccoli. Canned fish with bones is also a good source if you eat the bones too! Do not cut out dairy products from your diet unless advised to by a doctor.

## Fats and sugars

Essential fats (omega 3 and omega 6 fatty acids) are vital for our nerves to function properly and to keep our nails, hair and skin healthy. These are found naturally in foods in the groups above so you don't need any more. Keep added fats to a minimum – have just a scraping of reduced-fat olive or sunflower spread on bread, use the minimum sunflower or olive oil in cooking and avoid deep-frying. Also, reduce your intake of saturated animal fats (cut off meat fat, remove the skin from chicken, have skimmed or semi-skimmed milk, low-fat dairy products and so on).

Natural sugars are a good source of energy and are found in fruit, vegetables and grains. You don't need added sugar; it's loaded with calories with no added benefits. Keep it to a minimum, having sweet, sugary foods as occasional treats rather than filling up on them. When sweetening foods, I prefer to use honey as it is unrefined, it contains antioxidants and is sweeter than sugar, so you don't need so much.

## Drinks

It is vital that the body gets enough water, as it is the basis of every body function.

You need 2 litres/3$\frac{1}{2}$ pts/8$\frac{1}{2}$ cups of fluid a day. This doesn't have to be pure water; it's in every drink from milk to pure juice.

A few cautionary notes:

- Avoid sugary drinks – you don't need the empty calories.

- If you enjoy alcohol and can tolerate it, it should be limited to a maximum of 2–3 units a day for women and 3–4 for men, preferably less, and should not be counted as part of your water intake.

- Drinks containing caffeine – such as tea, coffee and cola – should also not be considered part of your water intake. Try not to drink too much; they act as a stimulant in moderation but are also likely to irritate your bowel. Also, having too much can stop your body from absorbing essential vitamins and minerals.

## NOTE FOR VEGETARIANS

IBS often causes flatulence, and legumes – dried peas beans and lentils – are prime culprits. But they are also a great source of vegetable protein and are important in a vegetarian diet. I do not recommend you cut them out of your diet completely.

Always soak them overnight before cooking and make sure they are cooked very thoroughly. The longer they are boiled, the less likely they are to cause flatulence. Alternatively, use canned ones but rinse them thoroughly before use and, ideally, mash or purée them for serving. If they do cause you problems, eat more eggs, tofu, dried soya protein and quorn instead. If you can tolerate cheese, then it, too, is an excellent source of protein.

# LEARNING HOW TO EXERCISE AND RELAX

I recommend you do some, what I call serious, exercise at least three times a week. That is playing a sport, going for a run, a brisk walk or a cycle ride, going for a 20-minute swim or doing a dance or aerobic exercise class. If you are not at all sporty, then rigorous activities like intensive gardening or even vacuuming the house (when you put your back into it!) can count. But, apart from that, you need to learn to do gentle exercise and relaxation every single day. That way you may well reduce the times you are in stressful situations, when an IBS attack is more likely.

It's a good idea to have some specific times each day when you do any of the following:

- Do yoga or pilates (you can buy books or DVDs or, preferably, join a class).

- Go for a slow swim.

- Go for a gentle jog.

- Take a stroll, preferably in a park or some other peaceful location. If you live in an inner city, there should still be some green spaces you can go to – even if it has to be the local cemetery or churchyard!

- Listen to tranquil music.

- Curl up in comfy clothes and read a good book.

- Watch a favourite DVD or video.

- Have a warm bath with relaxing essential oils.

- Once in a while treat yourself to a massage or an aromatherapy treatment at your local health spa.

Other activities to help increase your daily exercise:

- Take the stairs instead of the lift (elevator) or escalator.

- Get off the bus a stop early and walk the rest of the way.

- Park the other side of the car park from where you need to be, instead of the nearest possible space.

- Run upstairs instead of slowly plodding.

- Once a day, use the bottom stair or your doorstep as a 'step' and step up and down, putting your feet together after each movement 20 times.

## TENSION RELIEF EXERCISE

This can be done any time, any day when you feel your stress levels rising. Do it properly and I guarantee you will feel the tension melting away.

1. Stand erect but relaxed, feet slightly apart, arms by your side. Let your head drop on to your chest. Gently turn your head to the left so you are looking over your left shoulder. Gradually lift up your head, tilting it back so you look up to the ceiling, then roll it round to look over your right shoulder. Bring your head down and round so your chin rests on your chest again. Then lift it up to a normal forward-looking position. Repeat the other way.

2. Remain standing in the same position. Slowly shrug your shoulders, lifting them up under your ears. Drop them down suddenly. Repeat five times.

3. Remain standing in the same position, with your arms by your sides. Clench your fists tightly, hold for 5 seconds, then release.

4. Remain standing in the same position. Straighten your arms out to the sides so your elbows lock. Hold for 5 seconds, then let your arms relax and drop to your sides.

5. Remain standing in the same position. Tilt your head to one side down to the shoulder. Hold for 5 seconds, then straighten again. Repeat on the other side.

6. Remain standing in the same position. Push your stomach out as far as it will go. Hold for 5 seconds, then draw it in as tightly as you can. Hold for 5 seconds, then release.

7. Remain standing in the same position. Rise up on to your toes until you feel your calf muscles tighten. Hold for 5 seconds, then slowly return to standing normally.

8. Lie on the floor with your feet raised slightly off the floor, resting on the wall with your legs slightly bent. Push hard with your legs, as if trying to move the wall. Hold for 5 seconds, then relax.

9. Lower your legs so you are lying flat on the floor, arms by your sides. Close your eyes and breathe slowly and deeply. Relax every part of your body from your feet, through your spine, your arms, head and neck. Feel as if your body is melting into the floor beneath you. Lie like this for 2 minutes.

## SLEEP WELL, FEEL WELL

Follow these suggestions for ensuring a good night's sleep. Some are good old tried and tested ideas: others you may not have thought of:

### Before bed

- Have a warm bath with relaxing aromatherapy bath oils.

- Avoid caffeine or alcohol at bedtime: have a warm, milky drink or herbal tea instead.

- Wear comfortable night clothes.

- Listen to soothing, gentle music: avoid the loud, stimulating stuff.

- Don't watch disturbing television programmes or films or read anything unsettling.

- Don't eat fatty foods close to bedtime.

### The room and the bed

- Make sure the room is well ventilated but not draughty.

- Have a pot plant by the bed to 'balance' the air; a Christmas cactus is a good choice.

- Have the right amount of bedclothes – to be warm but not hot or cold.

- Have clean bedding on a regular basis.

- Warm the bed in winter before you get in.

- Have a comfortable pillow.

- Use a lavender fabric spray on your pillow to induce relaxation.

- Make sure the light is right for you – heavy curtains if you like the dark, lighter ones or slightly pulled back if you don't (and maybe a night light, if necessary).

## When in bed

- Use soft earplugs if your partner snores!

- Lie in the most comfortable position for you.

- Consciously relax your body (see the tension relief exercise number 9 on page 24).

- Breathe slowly, deeply and regularly.

- Try to clear your mind of all thoughts.

# YOUR SEVEN-DAY DIET PLAN

To start you off on your healthier diet, I have prepared a complete seven-day plan. This will get you into good habits and help you get used to eating well to alleviate and control your IBS. Once you have completed the plan, you can begin to experiment using the recipes in the main section of the book.

The diet plan is designed to suit whatever your lifestyle, and you can customise it as much as you like. For example, I have put the main meal at lunchtime but if it is more convenient for you to eat in the early evening, simply swap lunch and supper.

I have carefully planned each day to give a good balance of ingredients and nutrients. You can swap any day – or similar meal on a day – but just make sure that you still keep the balance and don't end up with, for instance, eggs for breakfast, lunch and dinner! I have made alternative suggestions for breakfast and supper dishes if you don't want to cook the recipe given. Any day that you don't want to follow the lunch recipe, have grilled (broiled), steamed or poached fish or white meat with any selection of vegetables or salad that you like.

I recommend at the end of breakfast (not the beginning) that you have a glass of pure fruit or mixed vegetable juice if you are not having a piece of fruit. If you can't tolerate pure juice, try watering it down. If it still causes problems, have a piece of diced fruit instead, or blend some fruit into a smoothie with milk and/or live bio yoghurt. Avoid juice drinks that are sweetened with sugar or artificial sweetener.

The plan incorporates a mixture of ready-prepared foods and home cooking as I know just what busy lives we all lead. We all use ready-prepared foods from time to time, but it is important not to live on ready meals as they tend to contain high amounts of salt, fat and sugar so won't help your problem one bit.

Make sure you have a glass of water with every meal and, ideally, at snack times too (it's the easiest way to ensure you drink enough fluids).

# EAT ACCORDING TO YOUR SYMPTOMS

Much of how you will manage your IBS will depend on whether you are suffering from diarrhoea or constipation. The meal plan is therefore marked, when necessary:

(D) if you suffer from diarrhoea
(C) if you suffer from constipation

If no symbol is shown it is suitable for everyone.

## DAY 1

| | |
|---|---|
| *Breakfast* | A bowl of porridge with milk and a trickle of honey |
| | A glass of pure fruit or mixed vegetable juice or a piece of fruit, chopped |
| *Mid-morning* | A rice cake with a scraping of peanut butter |
| *Lunch* | Mediterranean Vegetable Lasagne (see page 102) with Rocket and Cucumber Salad with Italian Buttermilk Dressing (see page 120) |
| | Apricot Almond Cooler (C) or a fruit low-fat live bio yoghurt |
| *Afternoon snack* | 1 Extra-good Oatcake (see page 146, or use bought) with a scraping of reduced-fat olive or sunflower spread and honey |
| *Supper* | Rich Barley, Tuna and Vegetable Soup (see page 55, or use a bought vegetable soup with a can of tuna added) |
| | A bread roll |
| | A fresh peach, peeled and chopped, or 2 canned peach halves in natural juice |

# DAY 2

| | |
|---|---|
| *Breakfast* | A slice of toast with a scraping of reduced-fat olive or sunflower spread, then<br>1 or 2 boiled eggs (D) or wholegrain cereal with a handful of raisins and a little milk (C)<br>A glass of pure fruit or mixed vegetable juice or a piece of fresh fruit, chopped |
| *Mid-morning* | A rice cake with a scraping of reduced-fat olive or sunflower spread and a scraping of Pear and Apple Spread (see page 155, or use a bought version from a health food shop), honey or peanut butter |
| *Lunch* | Grilled Salmon with Courgette Ribbons on Chive Mash (see page 83), with Saucy Wilted Spinach (see page 127)<br>Light Crème Brulée with Honey and Soft Fruit (see page 136) or a bought crème caramel |
| *Afternoon snack* | 1 Banana and Wheatgerm Muffin (see page 150) or 1 digestive biscuit (graham cracker) |
| *Supper* | Chicken Liver and Mushroom Pâté (see page 58, or use bought) with toast, a scraping of olive oil or sunflower spread, Seeded Fine-shred Coleslaw (see page 121, or use low-fat ready-made coleslaw with 5 ml/1 tsp toasted sesame seeds)<br>$^{1}/_{2}$ papaya (pawpaw), seeded and eaten with a spoon (add a squeeze of lime juice if you can tolerate it) |

# DAY 3

| | |
|---|---|
| *Breakfast* | Rolled Oats with Apple and Cinnamon (see page 38) or instant oat cereal with milk |
| | A glass of pure fruit or mixed vegetable juice or a piece of fresh fruit, chopped |
| *Mid-morning* | A small banana mashed with 60 ml/ 4 tbsp plain low-flat live bio yoghurt |
| *Lunch* | Dolcelatte, Courgette and Sweet Potato Pizza (see page 104) |
| | Peach and Almond Crumble (see page 139) or canned peaches |
| *Afternoon snack* | A handful of raw peanuts with raisins (C ) or a rice cake with a scraping of peanut butter (D) |
| *Supper* | Sardine Sizzle (see page 59) or canned sardines on toast served with some skinned, seeded and diced cucumber |
| | A small fresh mango, peeled, stoned (pitted) and diced or puréed |

## DAY 4

| | |
|---|---|
| *Breakfast* | Grilled Herby Flat Mushroom Bagel (see page 48) or plain stewed mushrooms on a toasted bagel<br>A glass of pure fruit or mixed vegetable juice or a piece of fresh fruit, chopped |
| *Mid-morning* | Rye crispbread with a scraping of peanut butter |
| *Lunch* | Chicken and Pak Choi Special Rice (see page 65)<br>Chocolate Sweet Soufflé Omelette (see page 138) or low-fat ice cream |
| *Afternoon snack* | A small banana |
| *Supper* | A small wedge of Edam cheese, some Extra-good Oatcakes (see page 146, or use bought) and a spoonful of Fresh Apple Relish (see page 156, or use bought chutney if you can tolerate it)<br>A fruit low-fat live bio yoghurt with complementing or contrasting fresh fruit to dip in |

# DAY 5

| | |
|---|---|
| *Breakfast* | A slice of toast with a scraping of reduced-fat olive or sunflower spread and Marmite<br>Dried Fruit Compôte with Bio Yoghurt (see page 40) or a can of fruit compôte in natural juice (C) or ½ papaya, peeled, seeded and diced with plain low-fat live bio yoghurt (D) |
| *Mid-morning* | A rice cake with a scraping of Pear and Apple Spread (see page 155, or use a bought version from a health food shop), peanut butter or honey |
| *Lunch* | Turkey Escalope with Sage and Mozzarella (see page 69), with Toasted Pepper Pasta (see page 128)<br>Pear and Marzipan Parcels (see page 137) |
| *Afternoon snack* | 1 digestive biscuit (graham cracker) |
| *Supper* | Chicken and Cashew Nut Soup (see page 56) or bought carrot and coriander soup<br>A bread roll<br>A plain low-fat live bio yoghurt with 5 ml/1 tsp clear honey |

# DAY 6

| | |
|---|---|
| *Breakfast* | Glazed Egg and Spinach Croustade (see page 49) (C) or Asparagus Light Fluffy Omelette (see page 50) (D) and a slice of toast or a bowl of instant oat cereal with a little milk and 5 ml/1 tsp honey<br>A glass of pure fruit or mixed vegetable juice or a piece of fresh fruit, chopped |
| *Mid-morning* | Rye crispbread with a scraping of reduced-fat olive or sunflower spread and Marmite |
| *Lunch* | Wild Mushroom, Chicken and Broccoli Risotto (see page 66)<br>Chocolate Mint Buttermilk Sorbet (see page 140) or low-fat ice cream |
| *Afternoon snack* | Almond and Raisin Oat Bite (see page 151) or a low-sugar fruit and cereal bar |
| *Supper* | Chilled Italian Prawn Platter (see page 54) or a ciabatta roll filled with prawns and mashed avocado<br>A small banana |

# DAY 7

| | |
|---|---|
| *Breakfast* | Toasted Millet and Oat Muesli (see page 39) or bought muesli, with a little milk<br>A glass of pure fruit or mixed vegetable juice or a piece of fresh fruit, chopped |
| *Mid-morning* | Rye crispbread with a scraping of reduced-fat olive or sunflower spread and Marmite |
| *Lunch* | Braised Duck with Baby Vegetables (see page 67)<br>Ginger Bread and Butter Pudding (see page 141) |
| *Afternoon snack* | A good handful of Light Savoury Popcorn (see page 154, or use unsweetened bought popcorn) |
| *Supper* | Sweet Spiced Lentil Soup (see page 57, or use bought lentil soup)<br>A bread roll<br>A fruit low-fat live bio yoghurt with complementing or contrasting fresh fruit to dip in |

# BASIC FOOD HYGIENE

A hygienic cook is a healthy cook – so please bear the following in mind when you're preparing food.

- Always wash your hands before preparing food.

- Always wash and dry fresh produce before use.

- Don't lick your fingers.

- Don't keep tasting and stirring with the same spoon. Use a clean spoon every time you taste the food.

- Don't put raw and cooked meat on the same shelf in the fridge. Store raw meat on the bottom shelf, so it can't drip over other foods. Keep all perishable foods wrapped separately. Don't overfill the fridge or it will run too warm.

- Never use a cloth to wipe down a chopping board you have been using for cutting up meat, for instance, then use the same one to wipe down your work surfaces – you will simply spread germs. Always wash your cloth well in hot, soapy water and, ideally, use an anti-bacterial kitchen cleaner on all surfaces too.

- Always transfer leftovers to a clean container and cover with a lid, clingfilm (plastic wrap) or foil. Leave until completely cold, then store in the fridge as soon as possible. Never put any warm food in the fridge.

- When reheating food, always make sure it is piping hot throughout, never just lukewarm. To test already made dishes, such as lasagne or a pie, insert a knife down through the centre. Leave for 5 seconds and remove. The blade should feel extremely hot. If not, heat a little longer.

- Don't re-freeze foods that have defrosted unless you cook them first. Never reheat previously cooked food more than once.

# NOTES ON THE RECIPES

- All ingredients are given in imperial, metric and American measures. Follow one set only in a recipe. American terms are given in brackets.

- The ingredients are listed in the order in which they are used in the recipe.

- All spoon measures are level: 1 tsp=5 ml; 1 tbsp=15 ml

- Eggs are medium unless otherwise stated.

- Always wash, peel, core and seed, if necessary, fresh produce before use.

- I have avoided using fresh onions or garlic, using granules instead as they are less likely to cause problems. However, if you can eat them fresh, substitute ½ a small finely chopped onion for 2.5 ml/ ½ tsp onion granules and ½ a small crushed garlic clove for 1.5 ml/¼ tsp garlic granules.

- Seasoning is very much a matter of personal taste. Taste the food as you cook and adjust to suit your own palate.

- Fresh herbs are great for garnishing and adding flavour. Pots of them are available in all good supermarkets. Keep your favourite ones on the window sill and water regularly. Jars of ready-prepared herbs, such as coriander (cilantro), and frozen ones – chopped parsley in particular – are also very useful. A few people find fresh herbs can cause symptoms – but this is rare. If so, substitute dried where fresh is called for in cooking (but use only about a third as much as the flavour is much more concentrated). Don't use dried for garnishing.

- All can and packet sizes are approximate as they vary from brand to brand. For example, if I call for a 400 g/14 oz/large can of tomatoes and yours is a 397 g can – that's fine.

- Cooking times are approximate and should be used as a guide only. Always check food is piping hot and cooked through before serving.

- Always preheat the oven and cook on the shelf just above the centre unless otherwise stated. This is not necessary if you have a fan oven.

- Use a reduced-fat olive or sunflower spread suitable for cooking and spreading instead of butter or ordinary margarine.

- Use skimmed or semi-skimmed milk, never full cream, and choose low-fat varieties of cheese, cream and yoghurt when appropriate.

# BREAKFASTS

Breakfast is an important meal for anyone, but especially an IBS sufferer. Your symptoms will be made much worse if you don't eat in the mornings. You don't have to cook a lavish breakfast every day; you can always have porridge, wholegrain cereal with milk, or a boiled, scrambled or poached egg on toast plus pure juice or a piece of fruit and decaffeinated coffee or tea. However, all the following make a fabulous start to the day and I thoroughly recommend them! I have avoided bacon as red meat can affect some people. If you can eat it, by all means enjoy a lean rasher or two, cooked with some mushrooms or with a poached or scrambled egg. It should be a treat though, not an everyday occurrence.

# Rolled Oats with Apple and Cinnamon

*You can also cook this in the microwave. Just use a non-metallic bowl and cook on High for the same amount of time. Even if you cannot usually drink a whole glass of apple juice without suffering, when used in small quantities in cooking – particularly with soluble fibre (oats in this case) – it should be fine.*

SERVES 1

*1 eating (dessert) apple, peeled, cored and diced*

*30 ml/2 tbsp apple juice*

*½ teacupful of rolled oats*

*1 teacupful of water*

*A good pinch of ground cinnamon*

*A pinch of salt*

To serve:

*Milk and 5 ml/1 tsp clear honey*

1 Put the apple and apple juice in a small non-stick saucepan. Bring to the boil, turn down the heat, cover and cook gently for 2 minutes.

2 Add all the remaining ingredients. Bring back to the boil, turn down the heat and simmer, stirring occasionally, for 5 minutes.

3 Turn into a bowl and serve with milk and the honey trickled over.

# Toasted Millet and Oat Muesli

*It's worth making a batch of this then you can store it in an airtight container to use any day you like.*

---

MAKES ABOUT 450 G/1 LB

---

*50 g/2 oz/¹/₂ cup millet grains*

*100 g/4 oz/1 cup rolled oats*

*50 g/2 oz/¹/₃ cup dried apricots*

*50 g/2 oz/¹/₃ cup raisins*

*50 g/2 oz/¹/₃ cup sultanas (golden raisins)*

*100 g/4 oz/1 cup toasted chopped mixed nuts*

*60 ml/4 tbsp dried milk powder (non-fat dry milk)*

To serve:

**Milk**

---

1 Put the millet in a non-stick frying pan. Heat, stirring, for about 3 minutes until the grains turn golden-brown. Tip out of the pan into a large container with an airtight lid straight away to prevent burning.

2 Add the rolled oats.

3 Snip the apricots into small pieces with scissors and add to the grains with all the remaining ingredients. Mix thoroughly, seal with the lid and store until ready to use.

4 Serve with milk.

# Dried Fruit Compôte
# with Bio Yoghurt

*It's not worth making this for one. Cook a batch and keep it in the fridge for use over the next few days. Alternatively, it can be frozen in portions for use as required.*

SERVES 4

*250 g/9 oz dried mixed soft fruit*

*300 ml/½ pt/1¼ cups water*

*1 cinnamon stick*

*Thinly pared zest of ½ small lemon*

To serve:

*Plain low-fat live bio yoghurt*

*60 ml/4 tbsp medium or coarse oatmeal*

1  Place all the ingredients in a saucepan.

2  Bring to the boil, reduce the heat, cover and cook very gently for 10–15 minutes until the fruit is tender. Discard the cinnamon and lemon zest.

3  Serve hot or cold in bowls with live bio yoghurt and a 15 ml/1 tbsp of oatmeal per serving.

# Toasted Oatmeal, Pear and Buttermilk Breakfast

*This is warming and utterly delicious. It's particularly enjoyable on a cold, grey winter's morning.*

| SERVES 1 |
|---|
| *30 ml/2 tbsp medium oatmeal* |
| *1 egg* |
| *75 ml/5 tbsp buttermilk* |
| *5 ml/1 tsp clear honey* |
| *15 ml/1 tbsp plain (all-purpose) or wholemeal flour* |
| *1 ripe pear, peeled, cored and diced* |
| *A small knob of reduced-fat olive or sunflower spread* |
| *A pinch of ground cinnamon* |

1 Heat a small non-stick pan. Add the oatmeal and stir until golden. Tip out of the pan and reserve.

2 Whisk the egg with the buttermilk, honey and flour in a small bowl.

3 Stir in the toasted oatmeal and the pear.

4 Heat the spread in the pan. Add the pear mixture and cook over a fairly low heat, stirring, until thickened and lightly scrambled, letting the mixture bubble – but only very gently.

5 Turn into a bowl, sprinkle with the cinnamon and serve hot.

# Blueberry Buttermilk Pancakes

*If you think this may be too much bother to make just for one, either share them with friends or family or store them, layered with non-stick baking parchment, and reheat them briefly in a non-stick pan before serving on other days.*

### MAKES 4

*50 g/2 oz/¹/₂ cup self-raising flour*

*50 g/2 oz/¹/₂ cup self-raising wholemeal flour*

*2.5 ml/¹/₂ tsp bicarbonate of soda (baking soda)*

*2.5 ml/¹/₂ tsp baking powder*

*A pinch of salt*

*60 ml/4 tbsp clear honey*

*2 eggs, beaten*

*120 ml/4 fl oz/¹/₂ cup buttermilk*

*120 ml/4 fl oz/¹/₂ cup milk*

*15 ml/1 tbsp sunflower oil, plus a little extra for greasing*

*75 g/3 oz/¹/₂ cup fresh or soft dried blueberries*

*5 ml/1 tsp grated lemon zest*

1　Mix together the dry ingredients in a bowl.

2　Add 15 ml/1 tbsp of the honey and all the remaining ingredients except the blueberries and lemon zest. Beat well to form a thick, smooth batter.

3　Mix in the blueberries.

4　Put the remaining honey and the lemon zest in a small pan and heat gently until runny. Remove from the heat and keep warm in a low oven.

5　Heat a small non-stick omelette pan and add a trickle of sunflower oil. Swirl round, then pour off the excess.

6　Add a quarter of the batter and spread it out to cover the base of the pan.

7 Cook until almost set and golden underneath and bubbles appear and pop on the surface. Flip over and cook the other side briefly. Slide out of the pan and keep warm in the oven while you cook the remainder.

8 Serve each pancake with a trickle of the lemon-flavoured honey.

# Traditional English Seeded Muffins

*These are divine cooked fresh for breakfast. Make the muffins the night before and store them in the fridge, then just griddle them before serving for breakfast. Alternatively cook them and store them in an airtight container and just split and toast to serve.*

MAKES 6

*100 g/4 oz/1 cup strong white bread flour*

*100 g/4 oz/1 cup plain (all-purpose) flour*

*30 ml/2 tbsp wheatgerm*

*2.5 ml/½ tsp salt*

*10 ml/2 tsp easy-blend dried yeast*

*15 ml/1 tbsp caraway seeds*

*15 g/½ oz/1 tbsp reduced-fat olive or sunflower spread*

*250 ml/8 fl oz/1 cup milk and water mixed*

*Oil for greasing*

*Cornflour (cornstarch) for dusting*

To serve:

*Reduced-fat olive or sunflower spread and honey*

1 Mix together the flours, wheatgerm, salt, yeast and seeds.

2 Heat the spread and milk and water together until warm but not hot.

3 Add to the flour mixture and mix with a wooden spoon until the mixture forms a very sticky dough, using your hands when it becomes too difficult with a spoon.

4 Cover the bowl with oiled clingfilm (plastic wrap) and leave in a warm place for about 45 minutes until the dough has doubled in size.

5 Knock back (punch down) the dough and divide into six equal pieces.

6 Oil a baking (cookie) sheet, then dust it with cornflour. With your hands and the work surface dusted with cornflour, shape the pieces into six balls. Place well apart on the baking sheet, cover loosely with oiled clingfilm and leave to rise for 30 minutes.

7 Heat a heavy-based griddle or frying pan until it feels hot when you hold your hand about 5 cm/2 in above it. Turn down the heat.

8 Place three muffins well apart in the pan and cook for 8 minutes on each side until pale golden with a thick white band round the middle. Wrap in a napkin while you cook the remainder.

9 Serve warm, pulled apart and spread with olive or sunflower spread and honey.

# Lightly Malted Linseed Breakfast Bread

*You can make this in a breadmaker if you prefer. Just make sure you add the fruit and seeds according to your manufacturer's instructions and cook the whole mixture on the basic programme.*

MAKES 1 SMALL LOAF

*225 g/8 oz/2 cups wholemeal flour, plus extra for dusting*

*100 g/4 oz/1 cup strong white bread flour*

*2.5 ml/¹/₂ tsp salt*

*15 ml/1 tbsp sunflower oil, plus extra for greasing*

*75 g/3 oz/¹/₂ cup mixed dried fruit (fruit cake mix)*

*25 g/1 oz/¹/₄ cup linseed*

*5 ml/1 tsp easy-blend dried yeast*

*15 ml/1 tbsp malt extract*

*175 ml/6 fl oz/³/₄ cup warm but not hot water*

*Beaten egg to glaze*

To serve:

*Reduced-fat olive or sunflower spread*

1  Mix the flours and salt in a large bowl.

2  Add the oil, fruit, linseed and yeast.

3  Blend the malt extract with the water and mix to form a soft but not sticky dough. Knead on a lightly floured surface for about 5 minutes until smooth and elastic.

4  Dust the bowl with a little flour and return the dough to it. Cover the bowl with oiled clingfilm (plastic wrap) and leave in a warm place for about 1 hour or until doubled in size.

5  Knock back (punch down) the dough, then shape it into a round and place on a floured non-stick baking (cookie) sheet. Cover loosely with oiled clingfilm and leave to rise for 30 minutes.

6 Preheat the oven to 220°C/425°F/gas 7/fan oven 200°C. Make several slashes in the top of the dough with a sharp knife and brush gently with the beaten egg to glaze.

7 Bake in the oven for about 30 minutes until risen, golden and the base sounds hollow when tapped. Transfer to a wire rack and leave to cool.

8 Serve sliced and spread with olive or sunflower spread. This loaf can be frozen.

# Grilled Herby Flat Mushroom Bagel

*If lean back bacon does not upset your stomach, you may enjoy a grilled rasher or two served alongside this. Have the other half bagel toasted with a scraping of spread and reduced-sugar marmalade (or save it to make the same breakfast in a couple of days).*

### SERVES 1

1 large flat mushroom

A knob of reduced-fat olive or sunflower spread

½ bagel

15g/½ oz/2 tbsp grated Edam cheese

15 ml/1 tbsp low-fat crème fraîche

5 ml/1 tsp chopped fresh parsley

5 ml/1 tsp snipped fresh chives

A good pinch of dried basil

Salt and freshly ground black pepper

1 Peel the mushroom and trim the stalk. Place, gills-side up, on foil on the grill (broiler) rack and smear with a little of the spread. Put the bagel half alongside. Grill (broil) for 2 minutes.

2 Meanwhile, mash the cheese with the crème fraîche, herbs and a little salt and pepper to taste.

3 Turn the bagel over (leave the mushroom) and grill for a further 1 minute. Remove the bagel and spread with a little olive or sunflower spread. Put on a plate and keep warm.

4 Pile the cheese mixture on to the mushroom. Grill for a further 2 minutes until the mushroom is soft and the cheese bubbling.

5 Transfer the mushroom to the bagel and serve straight away.

# Glazed Egg and Spinach Croustade

*This is a very elegant breakfast for when you have time to spoil yourself. It is extremely impressive if you are catering for others too.*

## SERVES 1

**100 g/4 oz thawed frozen or fresh leaf spinach, well washed**

**1 slice of bread**

**A scraping of reduced-fat olive or sunflower spread**

**1 egg**

**Salt and freshly ground black pepper**

**30 ml/2 tbsp low-fat crème fraîche**

1 Cook the spinach in a pan with no extra water for 5 minutes. Drain thoroughly and snip with scissors.

2 Meanwhile, cut the crusts off the slice of bread. Toast it on both sides under the grill (broiler). Remove the toast and put on a flameproof plate. Add a scraping of olive or sunflower spread. Keep the grill hot.

3 In a separate pan, poach the egg in gently simmering water with a pinch of salt added for 2–3 minutes or until cooked to your liking.

4 Put the spinach on the toast and add a good grinding of pepper.

5 Remove the egg from the pan with a draining spoon and slide on top of the spinach. Season the crème fraîche with a little salt and pepper and spoon over the egg. Flash under the grill until the top is glazed slightly. Serve hot.

# Asparagus Light Fluffy Omelette

*You can use mushrooms instead of the asparagus for a delicious variation. If you tolerate egg yolks, you can whisk them with 15 ml/1 tbsp water and fold them into the egg whites before cooking.*

---

SERVES 1

---

*2 large egg whites*

*Salt and freshly ground black pepper*

*A good pinch of dried mixed herbs*

*A little sunflower oil*

*½ × 212 ml/7½ fl oz/small jar of asparagus spears, drained*

To serve:

*A slice of toast*

---

1 Whisk the egg whites with a little salt and pepper and the herbs until stiff but not dry. They should still slide if the bowl is tilted.

2 Lightly grease a non-stick omelette pan with the oil. Add the egg whites and cook over a fairly gentle heat for about 3 minutes until golden underneath. Slide out of the pan on to a plate.

3 Lay the asparagus in the pan. Invert the omelette so the uncooked side is down, cook for a further 2 minutes, then tip out on to a plate and serve with toast.

# Smoked Haddock and Mushroom Topper

*This is best made for two people. If you are eating alone, store the other half in a covered container in the fridge and use it as a sandwich filling, with wholegrain bread and some lettuce.*

---

### SERVES 2

---

*1 small piece of undyed smoked haddock fillet, about 150 g/5 oz*

*45 ml/3 tbsp milk*

*1 × 295 g/10 oz/medium can of creamed mushrooms*

*A good pinch of dried oregano*

*A good pinch of pimentón*

*Salt and freshly ground black pepper*

*2 slices of bread*

*A scraping of reduced-fat olive or sunflower spread*

*A little chopped fresh parsley, to garnish*

1 Place the fish in a non-stick saucepan with the milk. Bring to the boil, reduce the heat, cover and simmer gently for 5 minutes until the fish flakes easily with a fork.

2 Using a draining spoon, transfer the fish to a plate. Flake the fish into small chunks, discarding the skin and any bones.

3 Stir the creamed mushrooms into the pan with the oregano and pimentón. Return to a gentle heat, stirring all the time, until piping hot.

4 Stir in the fish and season to taste.

5 Meanwhile toast the bread and add a scraping of spread. Put on plates, top with the haddock and mushroom mixture and sprinkle with the parsley before serving.

# Speciality Smoothie

*This is a good way to start the day for those who aren't breakfast fans. Ring the changes by adding other soft dried or fresh fruits with the banana and use other flavoured yoghurts to match or complement. It's fun to experiment!*

---

SERVES 1

---

**1 large banana**

**200 ml/7 fl oz/scant 1 cup milk**

**4 ready-to-eat dried apricots (the soft ones)**

**1 small carton of plain or apricot low-fat live bio yoghurt**

**30 ml/2 tbsp rolled oats or instant oat cereal**

**5 ml/1 tsp clear honey**

**30 ml/2 tbsp ground almonds**

---

1 Put all the ingredients in a blender. Run the machine until smooth and thick.

2 Pour into a very large glass and serve.

# LIGHT SUPPERS OR LUNCHES

These can be enjoyed in the evening or at lunch, if you prefer to have an early evening main meal. They are put together from ingredients that, hopefully, will help, not hinder your condition. If any of them contain trigger foods for you, simply substitute a similar ingredient.

# Chilled Italian Prawn Platter

*This looks and tastes wonderful and is so easy to prepare.*

---

**SERVES 1**

---

*1 × 125 g/4½ oz fresh Mozzarella cheese*

*A handful of frozen cooked, peeled king prawns (jumbo shrimp), thawed*

*1 small or ½ large avocado*

*1 slice of melon*

*A handful of black and green olives*

*A few fresh basil leaves*

*Freshly ground black pepper*

*About 15 ml/1 tbsp olive oil*

To serve:

*Ciabatta or other bread*

---

1 Holding the packet containing the cheese over the sink, snip off the end and pour out all the whey. Slice the cheese.

2 Dry the prawns on kitchen paper (paper towel).

3 Peel, stone (pit) and slice the avocado.

4 Peel and seed the slice of melon. Cut it in half lengthways to form two thinner wedges.

5 Arrange the cheese, prawns, avocado, melon and olives attractively on a platter. Tear the basil leaves into pieces and scatter over.

6 Add a good grinding of pepper and trickle the oil all over. Serve with ciabatta or other bread.

# Rich Barley, Tuna and Vegetable Soup

*There is no point in making soup for one. Make a pot and either share it with friends or family or cool, store in the fridge and have it over the next few days. The soup can also be frozen in portions, if preferred.*

## SERVES 4

*50 g/2 oz/generous ¼ cup pearl barley*

*1 carrot, coarsely grated*

*1 potato, coarsely grated*

*½ small swede (rutabaga), coarsely grated*

*900 ml/1½ pts/3¾ cups chicken stock, made with 1 stock cube*

*1 bay leaf*

*5 ml/1 tsp onion granules*

*1 × 185 g/6½ oz/small can of tuna, drained*

*Salt and freshly ground black pepper*

*30 ml/2 tbsp chopped fresh parsley*

To serve:

**Warm French bread**

1  Put the pearl barley, carrot, potato and swede in a saucepan. Add the stock, bay leaf and onion granules. Bring to the boil, reduce the heat, part-cover and simmer for 25 minutes.

2  Discard the bay leaf, then add the tuna, stir and simmer for another 5 minutes until the barley is tender. Season to taste.

3  Ladle into warm bowls, garnish with the parsley and serve with warm French bread.

# Chicken and Cashew Nut Soup

*This is so nutritious but is also so very good to eat! The nuts add texture as well as a rich creaminess.*

| SERVES 4 |
| --- |

**A knob of reduced-fat olive or sunflower spread**

**100 g/4 oz/1 cup raw cashew nuts**

**1 potato, diced**

**1 parsnip, diced**

**1 skinless chicken breast**

**2.5 ml/½ tsp ground cumin (optional)**

**1 litre/1¾ pts/4¼ cups chicken stock, made with 2 stock cubes**

**1 bouquet garni sachet**

**300 ml/½ pt/1¼ cups milk**

**Salt and freshly ground black pepper**

**15 ml/1 tbsp chopped fresh coriander (cilantro)**

To serve:

**Crusty bread**

1 Melt the spread in a large saucepan. Add the nuts, potato, parsnip, chicken and cumin, if using, and fry, stirring, for 2 minutes until lightly golden.

2 Add the stock and bouquet garni sachet, bring to the boil, reduce the heat and simmer for 20 minutes until the chicken and vegetables are cooked.

3 Lift the chicken out of the pan. Discard the bouquet garni.

4 Tip the contents of the pan into a blender or food processor and run the machine until smooth. Return to the pan.

5 Finely chop the chicken and add to the pan. Stir in the milk and season to taste. Stir in the coriander and reheat but do not allow to boil. Serve ladled into warm bowls with crusty bread.

# Sweet Spiced Lentil Soup

*This is so easy to make and is full of flavour. Soups are a good way to eat pulses and, being puréed, they are much easier to digest.*

SERVES 4

*2 carrots, chopped*

*½ small swede (rutabaga), chopped*

*5 ml/1 tsp ground coriander (cilantro)*

*150 g/5 oz/scant 1 cup red lentils*

*900 ml/1½ pt/3¾ cups chicken or vegetable stock, made with 1 stock cube*

*1 bay leaf*

*5 ml/1 tsp onion granules*

*Salt and freshly ground black pepper*

*15 ml/1 tbsp chopped fresh coriander (cilantro), to garnish*

1  Put all the ingredients in a pan. Bring to the boil, reduce the heat, part-cover and simmer for about 30 minutes until the lentils and vegetables are completely soft.

2  Liquidise in a blender or food processor. Return to the pan and heat through.

3  Taste the soup and re-season, if necessary. Ladle into warm bowls and garnish each with a sprinkling of chopped coriander.

# Chicken Liver and Mushroom Pâté

*This is very easy to make and is absolutely delicious served with hot toast and either the home-made Seeded Fine-shred Coleslaw on page 121 or a good-quality bought one made with low-fat mayonnaise (if you can tolerate it).*

### SERVES 4

*50 g/2 oz/¼ cup reduced-fat olive or sunflower spread*

*100 g/4 oz button mushrooms, sliced*

*1 potato, grated*

*350 g/12 oz chicken livers, trimmed of any sinews*

*5 ml/1 tsp garlic granules*

*5 ml/1 tsp onion granules*

*2.5 ml/½ tsp dried mixed herbs*

*15 ml/1 tbsp brandy*

*30 ml/2 tbsp low-fat crème fraîche*

*Salt and freshly ground black pepper*

To serve:

***Toast***

1  Melt half the spread in a saucepan. Add the mushrooms and cook, stirring, for 2 minutes until softened. Remove with a draining spoon and reserve.

2  Melt the remaining spread in the pan. Add the potato and cook, stirring, for 2 minutes until softened but not browned.

3  Add the chicken livers, garlic granules, onion granules and herbs and cook fairly gently for 4–5 minutes, stirring, until browned and just cooked but still soft.

4  Put the brandy in a soup ladle, warm it over a match or candle flame, then ignite. Pour over the chicken livers and stir until the flames subside.

5 Tip the mixture into a blender or food processor, add the crème fraîche and blend until smooth. Stir in the cooked mushrooms and season to taste.

6 Spoon into a small pot and level the surface. Leave until cold, then cover and chill.

7 Serve with toast.

# Sardine Sizzle

*This makes a tasty snack. Always mash the bones up as well as they are an excellent source of calcium.*

| SERVES 1 |
|---|

*1 × 125 g/4½ oz/small can of sardines in olive oil, drained*

*2.5 cm/1 in piece of cucumber*

*A handful of watercress, chopped*

*30 ml/2 tbsp low-fat crème fraîche*

*A few drops of Worcestershire sauce*

*Freshly ground black pepper*

*1 slice of bread*

1 Mash the sardines including the bones.

2 Peel the cucumber and halve it lengthways. Scoop out the seeds with a teaspoon and discard. Finely chop the flesh.

3 Work the cucumber, watercress, crème fraîche and Worcestershire sauce into the sardines. Season to taste with pepper.

4 Toast the bread on both sides under the grill (broiler). Pile the sardine mixture on top and return to the grill for 3–4 minutes or until the mixture is sizzling and hot. Serve straight away.

# Smoked Salmon Taramasalata

*This is a lovely, less oily version of the famous smoked cod's roe pâté. Enjoy it as a topping for a jacket-baked potato as well as a dip. The amount of lemon juice in this has been kept to the minimum – just enough to lift the flavour.*

### SERVES 2

**2 slices of white bread**

**100 g/4 oz smoked salmon trimmings**

**1.5 ml/¼ tsp onion granules**

**10 ml/2 tsp lemon juice**

**45 ml/3 tbsp sunflower oil**

**60 ml/4 tbsp boiling water**

**Salt and freshly ground black pepper**

To serve:

**Warm pitta breads, cut into strips**

1 Soak the bread in cold water for 2 minutes. Drain and squeeze out the excess moisture.

2 Put in a blender with all the remaining ingredients except the water and seasoning.

3 Run the machine, stopping and scraping down the sides as necessary until the mixture is smooth and thick. Blend in the boiling water, then season to taste.

4 Spoon into a small pot and serve with warm pitta bread strips.

# Pan Pesto Chicken Panini

*This is a delicious light meal. You can also add some fresh Mozzarella or a few baby spinach leaves if you like. Because pesto is pulverised and you are only having a small portion, it shouldn't cause problems.*

---

### SERVES 1

---

**1 panini, sandwich baton roll or a part-baked petit pain**

**15 ml/1 tbsp bought green pesto**

**1 slice of cooked chicken breast**

**1 baby cooked beetroot (red beet) (not in vinegar), sliced**

**Freshly ground black pepper**

**A little reduced-fat olive or sunflower spread**

1 Split the panini or roll lengthways, not right through.

2 Spread the inside with the pesto, then add the chicken and the beetroot slices. Season with pepper.

3 Spread the outside with a little olive or sunflower spread.

4 Heat an electric grill (broiler), add the panini and lower the lid but don't clip it shut. Cook for 3 minutes until golden-brown and stripy. Alternatively, cook in a griddle pan on the hob, pressing down with a fish slice, for about 2–3 minutes on each side. Serve hot.

# Mexican Tortilla Wedges with Cheese and Pimiento

*These are gorgeous warm any time of day. You can experiment with other fillings as long as you know you can tolerate them. Ham, in particular, is superb with the cheese!*

---

SERVES 1

---

**2 flour tortillas**

**40 g/1½ oz/⅓ cup grated Edam cheese**

**1 large or 2 small pimientos from a can or jar, drained and chopped**

**A good pinch of dried oregano**

**Freshly ground black pepper**

---

1  Lay one tortilla on a work surface.

2  Spread the cheese evenly over, then add the pimiento.

3  Sprinkle with the oregano, then a good grinding of pepper.

4  Top with the second tortilla and press down really well to flatten.

5  Heat a large, heavy non-stick frying pan. Turn the heat down low. Carefully transfer the tortilla to the pan and press a plate or saucepan lid on top to keep the tortilla as flat as possible. Cook gently for about 3 minutes until the cheese is melting and the base is turning a very pale golden-brown. Do not allow to brown too much.

6  Carefully turn over the tortillas, press down again and cook for a further 2 minutes. Slide out on to a plate and cut into small wedges. Eat with the fingers.

# Noodles in a Pot

*For some reason I cannot fathom, many people adore instant pots of flavoured noodles. Here you can have a highly nutritious version that will please your stomach as well as your tastebuds!*

---

### SERVES 1

---

*100 g/4 oz fresh prepared or thawed frozen Chinese stir-fry vegetables*

*1 slab of Chinese egg noodles or ¼ packet of rice (cellophane) noodles*

*2.5 ml/½ tsp chicken or vegetable stock powder*

*A pinch of garlic granules*

*A few drops of soy sauce*

---

1 Chop or snip the vegetables with scissors into much smaller pieces.

2 Put the noodles in a saucepan and just cover with boiling water. Stir in the stock powder and garlic granules. Bring to the boil and stir in the vegetables. Bring back to the boil and simmer for 5 minutes.

3 Drain thoroughly. Tip into a serving bowl and add a few drops of soy sauce to taste.

# WHITE MEAT MAIN MEALS

Red meat is much more likely to irritate IBS than white, so here is a selection of lovely chicken, turkey and duck recipes for you to enjoy with, hopefully, no side effects! I haven't included any game or rabbit recipes, but have recommended ones that would be suitable for their use.

It is very important that you eat the right foods and have the right balance. Your main meal should always include plenty of vegetables, either freshly cooked, frozen or canned. Don't skimp on them whatever you do. The addition of fresh and dried fruit to some of them is also a good way of getting more of your five-a-day and, because the fruit is cooked, it is unlikely to cause you problems. The serving suggestions are, of course, optional so you can substitute any vegetables that suit you and your palate. The recipes mostly serve one but are easy to increase if you are cooking for a family.

# Chicken and Pak Choi Special Rice

*If you can't get pak choi, you can use about ¼ head of spring (collard) greens instead. Cooking the stir-fry with a spoonful or two of water softens the vegetables slightly more than is usual for this way of cooking, which makes them more digestible for you.*

---

SERVES 1

---

*50 g/2 oz/¼ cup long-grain rice*

*10 ml/2 tsp sunflower oil*

*1 chicken breast, cut into thin strips*

*1 carrot, cut into thin strips*

*1 courgette (zucchini), cut into thin strips*

*1 head of pak choi, shredded*

*1.5 ml/¼ tsp Chinese five-spice powder*

*2.5 ml/½ tsp garlic granules*

*30 ml/2 tbsp water*

*A few drops of soy sauce*

---

1  Boil the rice in lightly salted water for 10 minutes or until just tender but still with some bite. Drain, rinse with cold water and drain again.

2  Heat the oil in a frying pan or wok. Add the chicken and stir-fry for 1 minute.

3  Add the vegetables, spice and garlic granules and stir-fry for a further 2 minutes.

4  Add the water, cover and cook for 4 minutes until the chicken is cooked through and the vegetables are just tender.

5  Stir in the rice and toss until hot. Season with a few drops of soy sauce to taste and serve.

# Wild Mushroom, Chicken and Broccoli Risotto

*This can be made with ordinary button mushrooms but the flavour won't be quite as good. The recipe also works well with rabbit.*

| SERVES 1 |
| --- |
| *10 ml/2 tsp sunflower oil* |
| *1 small skinless chicken breast, diced* |
| *50 g/2 oz wild mushrooms, sliced* |
| *50 g/2 oz/¹/₄ cup risotto rice* |
| *175 ml/6 fl oz/³/₄ cup chicken stock, made with ¹/₂ stock cube* |
| *1.5 ml/¹/₄ tsp garlic granules* |
| *A good pinch of dried thyme* |
| *Freshly ground black pepper* |
| *¹/₂ small head of broccoli, about 100 g/4 oz, cut into tiny florets* |
| *A little chopped fresh parsley* |

1 Heat the oil in a saucepan. Add the chicken and stir-fry for 1 minute.

2 Add all the remaining ingredients except the broccoli and parsley. Bring to the boil, turn down the heat and cook fairly gently, stirring occasionally, for 10 minutes.

3 Add the broccoli, stir and cook for a further 10 minutes until the liquid has absorbed, the rice is tender and the whole dish looks creamy. If necessary, add a dash of boiling water to bring it to the right consistency.

4 Spoon the risotto into a warm shallow soup plate and serve sprinkled with the parsley.

# Braised Duck with Baby Vegetables

*Do make sure you use a skinless duck breast or the result will be very fatty. This dish is based on a Victorian speciality but has far more veggies in it! You could use a skinned quail instead of the duck. If so, you may like to split it in half for easier cooking in the liquid. You can thicken the juices at the end with 5–10 ml/1–2 tsp cornflour, blended with a little water, if you like.*

SERVES 1

*1 skinless duck breast*

*1.5 ml/¼ tsp onion granules*

*5 baby potatoes, scrubbed*

*5 baby carrots, scrubbed*

*2 baby turnips, scrubbed and halved*

*150 ml/¼ pt/⅔ cup chicken stock, made with ½ stock cube*

*2.5 ml/½ tsp dried mint*

*1.5 ml/¼ tsp dried oregano*

*A pinch of grated nutmeg*

*Salt and freshly ground black pepper*

*1 small little gem lettuce, shredded*

*A handful of frozen peas*

1 Make a few slashes in the duck breast and rub with the onion granules.

2 Put the potatoes, carrots and turnips in a saucepan. Add the stock and stir in the mint, oregano, nutmeg and a little salt and pepper. Top with the duck.

3 Bring to the boil, reduce the heat, cover and simmer very gently for 20 minutes.

4 Stir in the lettuce and peas. Re-cover and simmer very gently for a further 5 minutes. Taste and re-season.

5 Transfer to a warm plate and serve hot.

# Chinese-style Duck Pilaf

*It's not worth making this for one. If you are eating alone, store the remainder in the fridge and have it cold as a salad or reheat it thoroughly the next day. The spring onions add colour and a nice sweet onion flavour. If you cannot tolerate them even when finely chopped, use 2.5 ml/½ tsp onion granules instead and garnish with a sprinkling of snipped fresh chives.*

---

### SERVES 2

*10 ml/2 tsp sunflower or olive oil*

*3 spring onions (scallions), finely chopped*

*1.5 ml/¼ tsp garlic granules*

*2.5 ml/½ tsp grated fresh root ginger*

*225 g/8 oz mini duck fillets, or 1 large skinless duck breast, cut into thin strips*

*100 g/4 oz/½ cup long-grain rice*

*300 ml/½ pt/1¼ cups chicken stock, made with ½ stock cube*

*5 ml/1 tsp clear honey*

*50 g/2 oz button mushrooms, sliced*

*1 red (bell) pepper, finely diced*

*50 g/2 oz/½ cup frozen peas*

*10 ml/2 tsp soy sauce*

*Freshly ground black pepper*

1  Heat the oil in a large, heavy-based shallow pan. Reserve a little of the green chopped spring onion tops for garnish, then add the remaining spring onions, the garlic granules, ginger and duck to the pan. Stir-fry for 3 minutes, then add the rice and stir until the grains are glistening.

2  Add all the remaining ingredients. Stir well, cover tightly, reduce the heat to as low as possible and cook very gently for 25 minutes.

3  Stir and check that everything is tender and the liquid has been absorbed. The rice should be moist but not wet. Taste and re-season if necessary.

4  Spoon the pilaf on to warm plates, garnish with the reserved chopped spring onion tops and serve.

# Turkey Escalope with Sage and Mozzarella

*If you can tolerate it, try spreading the turkey with a tiny spoonful of tomato purée before adding the cheese and herbs.*

| SERVES 1 |
| :---: |
| *1 turkey breast steak* |
| *Salt and freshly ground black pepper* |
| *3 slices of fresh Mozzarella cheese* |
| *1.5 ml/¹/₄ tsp dried sage* |
| *15 ml/1 tbsp olive oil* |
| To serve: |
| *Toasted Pepper Pasta (see page 128)* |

1  Put the turkey in a plastic bag and beat with a rolling pin or meat mallet to flatten. Remove from the bag and season with salt and pepper.

2  Lay the Mozzarella along the steak near one edge and sprinkle with the sage. Roll up firmly and secure with a wooden cocktail stick (toothpick).

3  Heat the oil in a frying pan. Add the turkey and brown quickly all over, then turn down the heat, cover the pan with foil or a lid and cook gently for about 8 minutes, turning once, until cooked through and the cheese is oozing out.

4  Transfer to a plate and pour the juices over. Serve with Toasted Pepper Pasta.

# Sautéed Chicken Livers with Rosemary and Redcurrant on Celeriac Mash

*Celeriac will keep well in the fridge, wrapped in clingfilm. The cut edge may go a bit brown but it can easily be trimmed off before cooking. The tomato purée adds depth of flavour but if you can't tolerate it, simply omit it.*

---

### SERVES 1

---

*100 g/4 oz chicken livers, trimmed of any sinews*

*2.5 ml/½ tsp onion granules*

*1.5 ml/¼ tsp dried rosemary, finely chopped*

*1 large potato, peeled and cut into small chunks*

*¼ head of celeriac (celery root), peeled and cut into small chunks*

*2 knobs of reduced-fat olive or sunflower spread*

*Salt and freshly ground black pepper*

*5 ml/1 tsp redcurrant jelly (clear conserve)*

*5 ml/1 tsp tomato purée (paste)*

*A little chopped fresh parsley*

To serve:

*Baby carrots*

1 Mix the chicken livers with the onion granules and rosemary and leave to marinate while preparing the mash.

2 Boil the potato and celeriac in lightly salted water for about 15 minutes or until really tender. Drain, reserving the cooking liquid, and mash thoroughly with one of the knobs of spread and a good grinding of pepper. Keep warm.

3 Melt the remaining spread in a small frying pan. Add the livers and cook, stirring, for 5 minutes until tender, browned but still soft.

**4** Add the redcurrant jelly, tomato purée and 75 ml/ 5 tbsp of the vegetable cooking water. Simmer fairly rapidly, stirring, for 3 minutes until slightly reduced. Season to taste.

**5** Spoon the mash on to a plate, make a nest in the middle and spoon in the liver mixture. Sprinkle with the parsley and serve with baby carrots.

# Chicken Tagine with Herbed Couscous

*This dish really benefits from the spring onion and a tiny bit of tomato purée. If they cause you problems, use 1.5 ml/ ¼ tsp of onion granules instead of the spring onion and simply omit the tomato purée. You can use rabbit or turkey instead of chicken.*

### SERVES 1

*1 skinless chicken breast, diced*

*1 spring onion (scallion), finely chopped*

*1 carrot, finely chopped*

*1 courgette (zucchini), diced*

*40 g/1½ oz/¼ cup raisins*

*1.5 ml/¼ tsp garlic granules*

*A good pinch of ground cinnamon*

*A good pinch of ground ginger*

*Salt and freshly ground black pepper*

*150 ml/¼ pt/⅔ cup water*

*5 ml/1 tsp chicken stock powder*

*2.5 ml/½ tsp dried oregano*

*50 g/2 oz/⅓ cup couscous*

*15 ml/1 tbsp chopped fresh parsley*

*5 ml/1 tsp tomato purée (paste)*

1  Put the chicken, vegetables, raisins, garlic granules, spices, a little salt and pepper, the water, stock powder and half the oregano in a saucepan. Bring to the boil, stirring. Reduce the heat, cover and cook gently for 10 minutes, stirring occasionally.

2  Meanwhile, put the couscous in a bowl and just cover with boiling water. Leave to stand for 5 minutes, then tip into a steamer or metal colander and stir in half the parsley and the remaining oregano.

3 Stir the tomato purée into the chicken. Put the steamer of couscous over the saucepan, cover and continue to cook for a further 5 minutes.

4 Fluff up the couscous with a fork. Taste the tagine and re-season, if necessary.

5 Spoon the couscous on to a serving plate. Spoon the chicken mixture on top and sprinkle with the remaining parsley before serving.

# Turkey Stroganoff on Buttered Broccoli Rice

*The broccoli rice goes well with any fish or poultry dish. For a creamier sauce, you can use low-fat crème fraîche instead of buttermilk, if you prefer. Try using rabbit or chicken instead of turkey too.*

## SERVES 1

*50 g/2 oz/¼ cup long-grain rice*

*100 g/4 oz head of broccoli, cut into tiny florets*

*2 good knobs of reduced-fat olive or sunflower spread*

*1 small turkey breast steak, cut into strips*

*5 mushrooms, sliced*

*1.5 ml/¼ tsp onion granules*

*15 ml/1 tbsp brandy*

*10 ml/2 tsp cornflour (cornstarch)*

*15 ml/1 tbsp water*

*90 ml/6 tbsp buttermilk*

*Salt and freshly ground black pepper*

*A little chopped fresh parsley, to garnish*

1 Boil the rice in lightly salted water for 10 minutes, adding the broccoli after 5 minutes. Drain thoroughly, return to the pan and toss with a good knob of the spread.

2 Meanwhile, heat the remaining spread in a small frying pan. Add the turkey and stir-fry for 3 minutes. Add the mushrooms and onion granules and continue to cook for 2 minutes until everything is cooked through.

3 Add the brandy and ignite. Shake the pan until the flames subside.

4   Blend the cornflour with the water. Stir into the
    buttermilk, then pour the mixture into the turkey.
    Bring to the boil and cook, stirring, for 1 minute.
    Season to taste.

5   Spoon the rice and broccoli on to a warm plate and
    spoon the stroganoff to one side. Sprinkle the
    stroganoff with the parsley and serve.

# Potato and Courgette Moussaka

*Traditionally this is served warm rather than hot as it really allows the flavours to develop. But that doesn't mean letting it get cold, then just warming it slightly (see Basic Food Hygiene, page 34). Again, I have used a little tomato purée in this. It can be omitted if you cannot tolerate even the tiniest amount.*

### SERVES 1

*1 potato, scrubbed and sliced*

*1 courgette (zucchini), sliced*

*10 ml/2 tsp olive oil*

*100 g/4 oz minced (ground) chicken*

*1.5 ml/¹/₄ tsp onion granules*

*1.5 ml/¹/₄ tsp garlic granules*

*120 ml/4 fl oz/¹/₂ cup chicken stock, made with ¹/₂ stock cube*

*5 ml/1 tsp tomato purée (paste)*

*1.5 ml/¹/₄ tsp ground cinnamon*

*1.5 ml/¹/₄ tsp dried oregano*

*30 ml/2 tbsp instant oat cereal*

*Salt and freshly ground black pepper*

*30 ml/2 tbsp plain (all-purpose) flour*

*150 ml/¹/₄ pt/²/₃ cup milk*

*A small knob of reduced-fat olive or sunflower spread*

*1.5 ml/¹/₄ tsp dried mixed herbs*

To serve:

*Feta Salad (page 123)*

1  Bring a large pan of water to the boil. Add the potato and boil for 2 minutes. Add the courgette and boil for a further 2–3 minutes until the vegetables are tender but still hold their shape. Drain, rinse with cold water and drain thoroughly again.

2  Heat the oil in a non-stick saucepan. Add the chicken, onion granules and garlic granules and cook, stirring, for 2 minutes until all the grains are separate.

3  Add the stock, tomato purée, cinnamon and oregano. Stir well and simmer gently for 2 minutes, stirring occasionally. Stir in the oat cereal and season to taste.

4  Blend the flour with the milk in a small saucepan. Stir in the spread and mixed herbs. Bring to the boil and cook for 2 minutes, stirring, until thickened and smooth. Season to taste.

5  Layer the vegetables and meat in a small ovenproof dish, finishing with a layer of vegetables.

6  Spoon the sauce over the layer of vegetables. Bake in a preheated oven at 190°C/375°F/gas 5/fan oven 170°C for about 40 minutes until the top is set and turning pale golden-brown. Leave to cool for 5–10 minutes, then serve warm with Feta Salad.

# Creamy Braised Poussin with Apples

*This is equally delicious with pheasant, quail or chicken too. Cook the jacket-baked potato at the same time as the poussin. You could use pear instead of apple for a variation.*

---

### SERVES 1

---

*1 poussin (Cornish hen)*

*A knob of reduced-fat olive or sunflower spread*

*1 eating (dessert) apple, peeled and sliced*

*Salt and freshly ground black pepper*

*2.5 ml/½ tsp onion granules*

*5 ml/1 tsp brandy*

*60 ml/4 tbsp cider or medium-dry white wine*

*75 ml/5 tbsp water*

*5 ml/1 tsp chicken stock powder*

*1 small bay leaf*

*10 ml/2 tsp cornflour (cornstarch)*

*15 ml/1 tbsp water*

*15 ml/1 tbsp low-fat crème fraîche*

*A little chopped fresh parsley, to garnish*

To serve:

*Jacket-baked potato and broccoli*

---

1 Remove as much skin as possible from the poussin and cut in half.

2 Place in a small flameproof casserole dish (Dutch oven) with all the remaining ingredients except the cornflour, water and crème fraîche.

3 Bring to the boil, cover tightly and transfer to a preheated oven at 180°C/350°F/gas 4/fan oven 160°F for 50–60 minutes.

4 Lift the poussin out of the pan and transfer to a warm plate. Keep warm.

5 Blend the cornflour with the water and stir into the juices. Bring to the boil, stirring, and cook for 1 minute. Stir in the crème fraîche and re-season if necessary.

6 Spoon the sauce over the poussin, sprinkle with the parsley and serve with a jacket-baked potato and broccoli.

# Chicken Satay

*Chicken satay, when bought, can be quite spicy. This version has all the goodness and rich flavour but none of the fire! If you can't tolerate lemon juice, use dry white wine instead.*

SERVES 1

**1 skinless chicken breast**

For the sauce:

**15 ml/1 tbsp smooth peanut butter**

**5 ml/1 tsp clear honey**

**5 ml/1 tsp lemon juice**

**5 ml/1 tsp soy sauce**

**1.5 ml/¼ tsp paprika**

**A pinch of ground cloves**

**30 ml/2 tbsp milk**

To serve:

**Spinach and Raisin Sticky Rice (see page 130)**

1 Cut the chicken into small dice. Thread tightly on two soaked wooden skewers.

2 To make the sauce, blend all the ingredients except the milk in a small saucepan. Heat through, stirring, until the peanut butter has melted. Stir in half the milk.

3 Lay the chicken kebabs on foil on the grill (broiler) rack. Spoon about a third of the sauce into a small container and use this to brush all over the chicken.

4 Grill (broil) the kebabs for about 6 minutes, turning once or twice, until golden and cooked through, brushing with the rest of the baste during cooking.

5 Stir the remaining milk into the remaining sauce and bring back to the boil, stirring all the time. Pour into a small serving dish.

6 Serve the kebabs with the sauce and Spinach and Raisin Sticky Rice.

# Warm Duck, Passionfruit, Asparagus and Broccoli Salad

*This is absolutely gorgeous any time but it is a bit decadent! You might like to serve it with a few boiled baby new potatoes too. Use the other half of the passionfruit to add an exotic flavour to a Speciality Smoothie (see page 52).*

SERVES 1

*100 g/4 oz head of broccoli, cut into tiny florets*

*50 g/2 oz baby asparagus spears, cut into short lengths*

*15 ml/1 tbsp olive oil*

*1 skinless duck breast*

*½ passionfruit*

*15 ml/1 tbsp buttermilk*

*5 ml/1 tsp clear honey*

*15 ml/1 tbsp water*

*Salt and freshly ground black pepper*

To serve:

*Warm crusty bread*

1  Cook the broccoli and asparagus in a steamer over a pan of boiling water for about 5 minutes or until tender. Remove the steamer from the pan.

2  Meanwhile, heat half the olive oil in a small frying pan and fry the duck for 3–4 minutes on each side until golden but still slightly pink in the centre. Remove from the pan and keep warm.

3  Remove the pan from the heat. Scoop the juice and seeds out of the shell of the passionfruit and tip into the pan with the remaining oil, the buttermilk, honey and water. Season lightly. Stir until blended.

4  Pile the broccoli and asparagus on to a warm plate. Slice the duck breast and arrange on top. Spoon the dressing over and serve with warm crusty bread.

# SEAFOOD MAIN MEALS

Fish is very digestible. Try to get a mixture of oily fish such as salmon, sardines and mackerel as well as white fish like cod, haddock and plaice. Not only is all fish good for you and can help to prevent heart disease, it is easy to prepare in a variety of ways. It may seem expensive at times but, remember, there is very little waste and, as it is so quick to cook, you use very little fuel too.

# Grilled Salmon with Courgette Ribbons on Chive Mash

*This is lovely with grilled tuna or swordfish too. It is so simple and easy to prepare.*

---

### SERVES 1

---

*1 large potato, peeled and cut into small chunks*

*1 courgette (zucchini), pared into strips with a vegetable peeler*

*A little olive oil*

*Salt and freshly ground black pepper*

*1 piece of salmon fillet, about 150 g/5 oz*

*2 knobs of reduced-fat olive or sunflower spread*

*15 ml/1 tbsp snipped fresh chives*

---

1 Put the potato in a pan well-covered with lightly salted water. Bring to the boil and cook for 3 minutes.

2 Meanwhile, put the courgette ribbons in a metal colander or steaming basket. After the 3 minutes, put the steamer over the potato pan, cover with a lid and steam for 4 minutes until the courgettes and potatoes are tender.

3 Meanwhile, brush a sheet of foil with a little oil on the grill (broiler) rack. Season the salmon lightly, then place skin-side up on the foil. Grill (broil) for 6 minutes until cooked through and the skin is golden. Do not turn over.

4 While the fish is cooking, drain the potatoes and return to the pan. Mash with a knob of the spread, the chives and a good grinding of pepper.

5 Pile the mash on to a plate, make a dip in the centre and add the remaining knob of spread so it melts into a pool. Pile the courgette ribbons alongside and top with the salmon, skin-side up.

# Double Haddock Kedgeree with Soft Boiled Egg

*This is a substantial dish but very pleasurable to eat! Buy the fish from a fishmonger so you can ask for the size of pieces you want. If you can't eat eggs, simply omit and add, if liked, some slices of fresh Mozzarella cheese on the top and allow to begin melting before you eat.*

### SERVES 1

*50 g/2 oz/¼ cup long-grain rice*

*1 egg, scrubbed under cold water*

*50 g/2 oz/½ cup frozen peas*

*1 small piece of smoked haddock fillet, about 75 g/3 oz*

*1 small piece of white haddock fillet, about 75 g/3 oz*

*45 ml/3 tbsp milk*

*15 ml/1 tbsp low-fat crème fraîche*

*1.5 ml/¼ tsp ground cumin*

*15 ml/1 tbsp chopped fresh parsley*

*Salt and freshly ground black pepper*

1 Boil the rice in lightly salted water for 10 minutes, adding the egg and peas for the last 4 minutes. Quickly remove the egg and plunge it into a bowl of cold water to prevent further cooking. Drain the rice and peas and return to the pan.

2 Meanwhile, cook the fish gently in the milk in a shallow pan, covered with a lid or foil, for about 5 minutes until the fish flakes easily with a fork. Remove from the milk and flake, discarding the skin and any bones.

3 Tip the flaked fish into the rice. Add 15 ml/1 tbsp of the cooking milk, the crème fraîche, cumin and most of the parsley. Heat gently, stirring, until well blended and piping hot.

4  Carefully shell the egg – don't forget it is soft-boiled (soft-cooked)! Pour the cold water away and put the egg back in the pan. Cover with boiling water for 1 minute (this will heat it through without further cooking).

5  Pile the fish and rice on to a warm plate. Lift out the egg with a draining spoon and put it on top. Cut it almost in half so the yolk trickles out. Sprinkle with the remaining parsley, season to taste and serve straight away.

# Almost Fat-free Fish and Chips with Cucumber Tartare

*Ordinary fish and chips is not good for IBS sufferers – far too much fat! This version is so much healthier for everyone. The flavour of the Cucumber Tartare is so good you won't mind not having vinegar!*

---

### SERVES 1

---

*1 cod or haddock fillet, about 150 g/5 oz, skinned*

*25 g/1 oz/½ cup fresh breadcrumbs*

*1.5 ml/¼ tsp dried thyme*

*5 ml/1 tsp onion granules*

*Salt and freshly ground black pepper*

*1 small egg white*

*100 g/4 oz frozen chips (not oven chips)*

*For the Cucumber Tartare:*

*2.5 cm/1 in piece of cucumber*

*30 ml/2 tbsp buttermilk*

*A good pinch of dried dill (dill weed)*

*A few drops of Worcestershire sauce*

To serve:

*Creamy Minted Mashed Peas (see page 125)*

---

1 Wipe the fish and remove any remaining bones.

2 Mix the breadcrumbs with the thyme, onion granules and some salt and pepper in a shallow dish. Lightly beat the egg white with a fork in a separate dish.

3 Dip the fish in the egg white, then in the breadcrumb mixture to coat completely. Place on a non-stick baking (cookie) sheet. Spread out the chips beside the fish.

4 Bake in a preheated oven at 220°C/425°F/gas 7/fan oven 200°C for 30 minutes until golden and cooked through.

5 Meanwhile, to make the sauce, peel the cucumber, cut it in half and scoop out the seeds with a teaspoon. Finely chop the flesh. Mix with the buttermilk, dill and Worcestershire sauce. Season to taste.

6 When the fish and chips are cooked, transfer to a warm plate and serve with the Cucumber Tartare and Creamy Minted Mashed Peas.

# Creamy Scallops

*This is based on a classic French dish but uses the little
queen scallops rather than the more expensive big meaty king
ones with the golden coral. It is a luxury to treat yourself
with! You can steam the asparagus in a metal colander or
steaming basket over the potatoes.*

---

### SERVES 1

---

*1 large potato, cut into small chunks*

*2 knobs of reduced-fat olive or sunflower spread*

*150 ml/¼ pt/⅔ cup milk, plus extra for mashing*

*Salt and freshly ground black pepper*

*6 button mushrooms, halved*

*100 g/4 oz queen scallops*

*30 ml/2 tbsp plain (all-purpose) flour*

*1.5 ml/¼ tsp onion granules*

*1 bay leaf*

*A pinch of dried mixed herbs*

*30 ml/2 tbsp low-fat crème fraîche*

To serve:

*Steamed baby asparagus spears*

---

1　Boil the potato in lightly salted water for about
　6 minutes or until tender. Drain and mash with a knob
　of spread and about 15 ml/1 tbsp milk until creamy.
　Season with pepper.

2　Meanwhile, melt the remaining spread in a small non-
　stick saucepan. Add the mushrooms and scallops and
　cook for 2 minutes, stirring. Remove from the pan with
　a draining spoon.

3　Remove the pan from the heat. Blend the flour into the
　cooking juices, then stir in the milk until smooth. Add
　the onion granules, bay leaf and herbs. Bring to the
　boil and cook for 2 minutes, stirring, until thickened
　and smooth.

**4** Stir in the crème fraîche and season to taste. Remove the bay leaf and add the scallops and mushrooms to the sauce. Turn into a flameproof dish.

**5** Spoon the mashed potato on top and rough up with a fork. Place under a preheated grill (broiler) for about 5 minutes until golden on top. Serve hot with steamed baby asparagus spears.

# Red Mackerel with Crushed Turnips, Peas and Potatoes

*Pimentón is worth having in the cupboard as it can be used with lots of food to give a lovely smoky flavour.*

---
SERVES 1
---

**1 fresh mackerel, cleaned**

**1.5 ml/¼ tsp ground paprika**

**1.5 ml/¼ tsp pimentón**

**1.5 ml/¼ tsp ground cumin**

**10 ml/2 tsp olive oil**

**A pinch of salt**

**1 potato, peeled and cut into chunks**

**1 turnip, peeled and cut into chunks**

**50 g/2 oz/½ cup frozen peas**

**A small knob of reduced-fat olive or sunflower spread**

**A sprig of parsley, to garnish**

---

1 Rinse the fish in cold water and pat dry on kitchen paper (paper towels). Make several slashes on both sides of the fish.

2 Mix the spices with the oil and salt. Spread over both sides of the fish, rubbing it well into the slits. Lay the fish on a sheet of foil on the grill (broiler) rack. Grill (broil) the fish for 5 minutes on each side until golden and cooked through.

3 Meanwhile, boil the potato and turnip in lightly salted water for 5 minutes. Add the peas and cook for a further 3–4 minutes until everything is tender.

4 Drain the vegetables and return to the pan. Add the spread and crush the vegetables with a fork, mixing and turning but not mashing them to a purée – they should still have some texture.

5 Pile the crushed vegetables on to a warm plate and lay the fish alongside. Garnish with the parsley and serve.

# Warm Tuna, Beetroot and Baby Potato Salad

*This is a lovely all-in-one meal. Try it with canned salmon or even pilchards in olive oil (thoroughly drained) too. It's cheaper to use this size can of tuna than a very tiny one, so store the rest of the fish in a covered container – not in the can – in the fridge for another meal.*

---

### SERVES 1

*5 baby potatoes, scrubbed and halved*

*2 baby turnips, peeled and quartered*

*2.5 cm/1 in piece of cucumber*

*2 cooked baby beetroot (red beets) (not in vinegar), diced*

*30 ml/2 tbsp low-fat crème fraîche*

*A good pinch of garlic or onion granules*

*A few drops of Worcestershire sauce*

*Salt and freshly ground black pepper*

*½ × 185 g/6½ oz/small can of tuna, drained*

To serve:

*A multigrain bread roll*

---

1 Boil the potatoes and turnips in lightly salted water for about 8 minutes or until tender. Drain and return to the pan.

2 Peel and halve the cucumber. Scoop out the seeds with a teaspoon and dice the flesh. Add to the potatoes and turnips with the beetroot.

3 Mix the crème fraîche with the garlic or onion granules, a few drops of Worcestershire sauce and salt and pepper to taste.

4 Add the tuna to the vegetables, then the dressing. Toss gently and serve while still warm with a multigrain bread roll.

# Penne with King Prawns

*You do need to buy the raw king prawns to get the best flavour for this dish. Experiment with mixed seafood instead of all prawns too.*

### SERVES 1

*5 ml/1 tsp olive oil*

*1 wedge of celeriac (celery root), finely diced*

*1 carrot, finely diced*

*75 g/3 oz penne pasta*

*300 ml/½ pt/1¼ cups fish stock, made with ½ stock cube*

*1 pimiento cap from a can or jar, diced*

*1.5 ml/¼ tsp onion granules*

*1.5 ml/¼ tsp garlic granules*

*1.5 ml/¼ tsp dried oregano*

*100 g/4 oz frozen raw shelled king prawns (shrimp)*

*50 g/2 oz/½ cup frozen peas*

*Salt and freshly ground black pepper*

*A little chopped fresh parsley*

To serve:

*French bread and Rocket and Cucumber Salad with Italian Buttermilk Dressing (see page 120)*

1  Heat the oil in a shallow pan. Add the celeriac and carrot and cook, stirring, for 2 minutes.

2  Stir in the penne until glistening, then add the stock, pimiento, onion granules, garlic granules and oregano. Bring to the boil, stirring, then turn down the heat, cover and cook gently for 10 minutes, stirring occasionally.

3  Add the prawns and peas and season to taste. Stir, re-cover and cook gently for a further 10 minutes, stirring occasionally, until the pasta is tender and has absorbed the liquid and the prawns are pink.

**4** Taste and re-season if necessary. Sprinkle with the parsley and serve with French bread and Rocket and Cucumber Salad with Italian Buttermilk Dressing.

# Stuffed Plaice with Pesto and Pine Nut Spaghetti

*This has a lovely flavour but is so easy to prepare. Because pesto is puréed, it should not cause you any problems.*

---

### SERVES 1

---

*1 large plaice fillet, skinned, if preferred*

*15 ml/1 tbsp pine nuts*

*¼ × 500 g/18 oz packet of spaghetti*

*15 ml/1 tbsp pesto sauce from a jar*

*15 g/½ oz/¼ cup fresh breadcrumbs*

*75 ml/5 tbsp fish or chicken stock,
made with ¼ stock cube*

*30 ml/2 tbsp dry white wine*

*Salt and freshly ground black pepper*

*15 ml/1 tbsp low-fat crème fraîche*

*5 ml/1 tsp olive oil*

To serve:

*Avocado Salad (see page 122)*

---

1 Cut the plaice in half to make two smaller fillets.

2 Put the pine nuts in a saucepan and heat, tossing, until golden. Tip out of the pan and reserve.

3 Using the same pan, boil the spaghetti in lightly salted water for 10 minutes or according to the packet directions. Drain and return to the pan.

4 Meanwhile, mix the pesto with the breadcrumbs. Lay the plaice fillets on a board, flesh-side down, and spread with the pesto mixture. Roll up, starting at the thick end.

5 Place in a small shallow pan with the tail ends down. Add the stock, wine, a sprinkling of salt and a good grinding of pepper. Bring to the boil, cover with a lid or foil and cook gently for 5 minutes.

6 Remove the lid and lift the fish out of the pan. Keep warm. Turn up the heat and boil the cooking juices for 2 minutes until reduced by half. Stir in the crème fraîche, taste and re-season if necessary.

7 Add the oil to the cooked spaghetti with the pine nuts and a good grinding of pepper. Toss over a gentle heat until glistening and hot through.

8 Transfer the spaghetti to a warm plate. Top with the fish and the sauce and serve with Avocado Salad.

# Cod Wrapped in Cabbage with Prawn Sauce

*This is an elegant dish to serve for a special occasion. It can easily be made for more people but is a real treat if you are eating alone.*

---

### SERVES 1

*1 large cabbage leaf*

*1 rectangular frozen cod steak, thawed*

*Salt and freshly ground black pepper*

*45 ml/3 tbsp dry white wine*

*45 ml/3 tbsp water*

*2.5 ml/½ tsp vegetable stock powder*

For the sauce:

*15 ml/1 tbsp plain (all-purpose) flour*

*75 ml/5 tbsp milk*

*A very small knob of reduced-fat olive or sunflower spread, plus extra for greasing*

*A good pinch of dried dill (dill weed)*

*25 g/1 oz cooked, peeled prawns (shrimp), thawed if frozen*

*15 ml/1 tbsp chopped fresh parsley*

To serve:

*Baby new potatoes*

---

1 Trim away any thick stump from the cabbage leaf. Blanch the leaf in boiling water for 3 minutes, then drain, rinse with cold water and drain again. Pat dry on kitchen paper (paper towels).

2 Lay the leaf outer-side down on a board. Put the cod in the centre and season lightly. Wrap up and place in a small, shallow pan, flaps down. Add the wine, water and stock powder.

3 Bring to the boil, then cover tightly with a lid or foil. Turn down the heat to very low and cook gently for 20 minutes or until the cabbage is tender.

4 Meanwhile, to make the sauce, blend the flour and milk in a small saucepan. Add the spread. Bring to the boil and cook for 2 minutes, stirring, until thickened and smooth. Stir in the dill, prawns and parsley and season to taste. Heat through gently.

5 Carefully lift the cabbage-wrapped cod out of the pan and transfer to a warm plate. Boil the juices until reduced by half and stir into the prawn sauce. Spoon the sauce over the cod and serve with baby new potatoes.

# Aubergine, Smoked Salmon and Mozzarella Layer

*This may sound decadent but it uses only two small slices of smoked salmon! Mixing just a dash of tomato purée with mashed carrots gives a lovely tangy sweet flavour but with none of the problems you might get if you used all tomatoes.*

---

### SERVES 1

---

*½ aubergine (eggplant)*

*15 ml/1 tbsp olive oil*

*1 cooked carrot or 4 small canned carrots*

*5 ml/1 tsp tomato purée (paste)*

*2 small, thin slices of smoked salmon*

*1 × 125 g/4½ oz fresh Mozzarella cheese, drained and sliced*

*15 ml/1 tbsp chopped fresh basil*

*Salt and freshly ground black pepper*

*30 ml/2 tbsp water*

To serve:

***Crusty bread and Warm Celeriac and Courgette Salad (see page 126)***

---

1 Trim the aubergine and cut it lengthways into in two slices. Brush both slices lightly all over with olive oil.

2 Heat a griddle pan and cook the slices for about 2 minutes on each side until cooked and stripy. Alternatively, cook in an electric grill for 2 minutes in all.

3 Mash the carrot with the tomato purée.

4 Place one aubergine slice, cut-side up, in a shallow flameproof dish. Lay a slice of salmon on top, folded to fit.

5 Spread the carrot mixture on top, then add the other slice of salmon, folded to fit.

6  Top with the Mozzarella slices, then the basil. Season with salt and pepper.

7  Lay the second slice of aubergine on top and spoon the water around. Cover the dish with foil.

8  Bake in a preheated oven at 220°C/425°F/gas 7/fan oven 200°C for 15 minutes until cooked through and the cheese has melted. Transfer to a warm plate and serve with crusty bread and Warm Celeriac and Courgette Salad.

# VEGETARIAN MAIN MEALS

Being a vegetarian with IBS can be tricky as so many of your staples can cause problems. As I've said before, the key is cutting up vegetables small, or mashing, grating or cooking them thoroughly, to reduce possible reaction.

Here are some delicious dishes that should cause you few or no problems at all. Remember to always rinse canned pulses before using and mash or purée them if you can't tolerate them whole. Don't cut them out completely unless you absolutely have to, as they are an important source of many essential nutrients – especially protein – for vegetarians.

# Green Tagliatelle with Spinach and Walnut Sauce

*Spinach and walnuts go surprisingly well together. You shouldn't have a problem with the Parmesan in this but, if you can't tolerate it, you could add a little celery salt to taste instead and omit the shavings for garnish.*

## SERVES 1

*75 g/3 oz green tagliatelle*

*100 g/4 oz frozen leaf spinach, thawed*

*60 ml/4 tbsp low-fat crème fraîche*

*5 ml/1 tsp grated Parmesan cheese*

*15 ml/1 tbsp finely chopped walnuts*

*Salt and freshly ground black pepper*

*1.5 ml/¼ tsp dried mixed herbs*

*15 ml/1 tbsp fresh Parmesan shavings (optional)*

1 Cook the pasta according to the packet directions. Drain.

2 Add the spinach to the pasta pan and cook for 2 minutes, stirring. Drain and squeeze out as much moisture as possible, then tip back into the pan. Snip with scissors to chop.

3 Stir in the crème fraîche, grated Parmesan, walnuts, a little seasoning and the herbs. Heat, stirring, until piping hot.

4 Add the cooked pasta and toss thoroughly.

5 Pile on to a warm plate and scatter some fresh Parmesan shavings over, if liked.

# Mediterranean Vegetable Lasagne

*This is a lovely change from a meat, bean or fish pasta layer. If you can tolerate tomatoes, you can add some passata instead of or as well as the wine and bubble slightly longer to reduce.*

### SERVES 1

1 red (bell) pepper

1 small or ½ large aubergine (eggplant)

15 ml/1 tbsp olive oil

1 courgette (zucchini), trimmed and chopped

1.5 ml/¼ tsp garlic granules

1.5 ml/¼ tsp dried oregano

30 ml/2 tbsp red wine

30 ml/2 tbsp water

1.5 ml/¼ tsp vegetable stock powder

Salt and freshly ground black pepper

30 ml/2 tbsp plain (all-purpose) flour

150 ml/¼ pt/⅔ cup milk

A knob of reduced-fat olive or sunflower spread

25 g/1 oz/¼ cup grated Edam cheese

3 sheets of no-need-to-precook lasagne

To serve:

**Rocket and Cucumber Salad with Italian Buttermilk Dressing (see page 120)**

1  Put the red pepper and aubergine under the grill (broiler). Grill (broil), turning occasionally, for about 15 minutes until blackened all over.

2  Pop them in a plastic bag and leave until cool enough to handle, then peel off the blackened skins. Remove the seeds and stalk from the pepper and the stalk from the aubergine. Chop the flesh.

3 Heat the oil in a saucepan. Add the courgette and fry for 2 minutes, stirring. Add the chopped pepper and aubergine, the garlic granules, oregano, wine, water, stock and a sprinkling of salt and pepper. Bring to the boil, reduce the heat, part-cover and simmer gently for 5 minutes until most of the liquid has been absorbed.

4 Meanwhile, blend the flour with the milk in a small saucepan using a wire whisk. Add the knob of spread. Bring to the boil, whisking all the time, until thick and smooth. Stir in the cheese and season to taste.

5 Spread a tiny bit of the sauce on the base of a small shallow dish, large enough to take a lasagne sheet.

6 Put a lasagne sheet on top, then half the vegetable mixture. Repeat the layers of lasagne and vegetables, finishing with the last lasagne sheet.

7 Spoon the remaining sauce over. Bake in a preheated oven at 190°C/375°F/gas 5/fan oven 170°C for 35 minutes until tender and golden. Serve with Rocket and Cucumber Salad with Italian Buttermilk Dressing.

# Dolcelatte, Courgette and Sweet Potato Pizza

*If you can't eat blue cheese, use silken tofu and flavour it with a few drops of Worcestershire sauce and a sprinkling of garlic granules. If the whole pizza is too much for one meal, the rest tastes really good cold for lunch the next day!*

### SERVES 1

1 × 225 g/10 oz packet of pizza base mix

120 ml/4 fl oz/½ cup hand-hot water

Flour for dusting

15 ml/1 tbsp olive oil, plus extra for greasing and drizzling

1 small uncooked beetroot (red beet), diced

1 courgette (zucchini), diced

1 small sweet potato, diced

50 g/2 oz/½ cup Dolcelatte, crumbled

1 × 125 g/4½ oz fresh Mozzarella cheese, drained and grated

2.5 ml/½ tsp dried sage or 4 fresh leaves, chopped

1.5 ml/¼ tsp onion granules

Freshly ground black pepper

1  Mix the pizza dough with enough of the hand-hot water to form a soft but not sticky dough. Knead gently on a lightly floured surface for 5 minutes until smooth and elastic. Alternatively, make it in a food processor and, once the dough has formed, run the machine for 1 minute to knead.

2  Roll out to a 23 cm/9 in round and place on an oiled pizza plate or baking (cookie) sheet. Leave in a warm place while preparing the topping.

**3** Put the beetroot, courgette and sweet potato in a saucepan. Add the olive oil and toss well using your hands. Cook over a high heat until beginning to sizzle, then turn down the heat, cover with a lid or foil and cook for about 12 minutes, stirring occasionally, until the vegetables are tender.

**4** Scatter the cooked vegetables over the dough, then add the cheeses, sage, onion granules and a good grinding of pepper. Bake in a preheated oven at 220°C/425°F/gas 7/fan oven 200°C for about 20 minutes or until golden round the edges and the cheese is melted and bubbling.

# Tofu, Courgette and Mushroom Kebabs with Hummus Sauce

*Cooking this for two uses up all the ingredients. You can halve the quantity, then store the remaining tofu and hummus in the fridge for another day. The amount of lemon juice in the bought hummus should not be a problem. But if you are ultra-sensitive, you could use the yoghurt dressing that is served with the Soya Rissoles on page 110 instead. For strict vegetarians, make sure the Worcestershire sauce is suitable.*

---

### SERVES 2

*2 courgettes (zucchini), each cut into 6 chunks*

*12 button mushrooms*

*1 block of firm tofu, drained and cut into 12 cubes*

*5 ml/1 tsp sunflower oil*

*15 ml/1 tbsp Worcestershire sauce*

*10 ml/2 tsp soy sauce*

*1 × 170 g/6 oz/small tub of low-fat hummus*

*60 ml/4 tbsp milk*

*15 ml/1 tbsp chopped fresh parsley*

To serve:

*Wild rice mix*

---

1 Bring a small pan of water to the boil, add the courgettes and mushrooms and boil for 2 minutes. Drain, rinse with cold water and drain again.

2 Thread the courgettes, mushrooms and tofu cubes on four metal skewers.

3 Mix together the oil, Worcestershire sauce and soy sauce and brush all over the kebabs.

4 Lay the kebabs on foil on the grill (broiler) rack. Grill (broil) for about 8 minutes, turning occasionally and brushing with any remaining baste, until cooked through and turning lightly golden.

5 Meanwhile, mix the hummus with the milk and parsley in a small saucepan. Heat gently until piping hot, but do not allow to boil.

6 Serve the kebabs on a bed of wild rice mix with the sauce trickled over.

# Quorn, Carrot and Mushroom Pie

*Filo pastry is very low in fat so is the ideal 'wrapper' for loads of savoury and sweet fillings. Try it baked into little tartlet cases and filled with the vegetable mixture for Mediterranean Vegetable Lasagne on page 102.*

SERVES 1

75 g/3 oz quorn pieces

1.5 ml/¼ tsp onion granules

1 carrot, finely diced

3 mushrooms, sliced

150 ml/¼ pt/⅔ cup vegetable stock,
made with ½ stock cube

1 small bay leaf

Salt and freshly ground black pepper

15 ml/1 tbsp plain (all-purpose) flour

60 ml/4 tbsp cold water

1 sheet of filo pastry (paste)

A little sunflower oil

To serve:

Cabbage with Walnuts (see page 133)

1  Put the quorn, onion granules, carrot, mushrooms, stock, bay leaf and a little salt and pepper in a saucepan. Bring to the boil, reduce the heat, cover and simmer gently for 10 minutes until everything is tender.

2  Blend the flour with the water, stir into the mixture, bring back to the boil and cook for 2 minutes, stirring. Tip into an individual deep pie (or similar) dish. Cover with foil.

3 Brush the filo with a very little oil. Fold in half and brush with a little more oil. Crumple slightly as you would a piece of paper, so it is about the size of the top of the pie dish. Place on a lightly oiled baking (cookie) sheet.

4 Bake the pastry with the dish of pie filling alongside in a preheated oven at 190°C/375°F/gas 5/fan oven 170°C for 5 minutes or until the pastry is crisp and golden on top. Carefully transfer the pastry to the top of the pie. Serve with Cabbage with Walnuts.

# Mild-spiced Soya Rissoles with Minted Yoghurt Dressing

*These delicious rissoles can be bound with 1 large egg white if you can't tolerate egg yolks. They taste surprisingly meaty and substantial. I make loads of dressing to dip the naan bread into. Try it with the Fresh Apple Relish on page 156 too.*

---

SERVES 2

---

For the dressing:

*150 ml/¼ pt/⅔ cup plain low-fat live bio yoghurt*

*2.5 ml/½ tsp garlic granules*

*10 ml/2 tsp dried mint*

*7.5 cm/3 in piece of cucumber, peeled, seeded and finely chopped*

*A few salad leaves and slices of avocado, to garnish*

For the rissoles:

*25 g/1 oz/¼ cup dried soya mince*

*½ small sweet potato, grated*

*5 ml/1 tsp garam masala*

*2.5 ml/½ tsp onion granules*

*50 g/2 oz/1 cup fresh breadcrumbs*

*30 ml/2 tbsp chopped fresh coriander (cilantro) (optional)*

*1 small egg, beaten*

*Salt and freshly ground black pepper*

*25 g/1 oz/¼ cup dried breadcrumbs*

*A little sunflower oil for brushing*

To serve:

*Plain naan bread and Warm Celeriac and Courgette Salad (see page 126)*

1 To make the dressing, mix together all the ingredients in a bowl. Chill.

2 To make the rissoles, put the soya protein in a bowl. Just cover with boiling water and leave to stand for at least 1 minute, then drain well.

3 Mix the soya with all the remaining ingredients except the dried breadcrumbs, seasoning the mixture well.

4 Squeeze the mixture well together, then shape into four round cakes and coat in the dried breadcrumbs. Chill, if time, before cooking.

5 Place the rissoles on foil on a grill (broiler) rack and brush all over with a little oil. Grill (broil) for about 5 minutes on each side until golden and cooked through.

6 Transfer the rissoles to warm plates and serve with the dressing, naan bread and Warm Celeriac and Courgette Salad.

# Nut Roast-stuffed Pepper with Carrot Gravy

*You may find you have too much gravy for one. If so, cool it and store it in an airtight container in the fridge for another meal or freeze it for future use.*

---

### SERVES 1

---

**50 g/2 oz/½ cup raw cashew nuts, chopped**

**25 g/1 oz/½ cup fresh breadcrumbs**

**1.5 ml/¼ tsp onion granules**

**5 ml/1 tsp soy sauce**

**A good pinch of dried oregano**

**A knob of reduced-fat olive or sunflower spread**

**2.5 ml/½ tsp Marmite or other yeast extract**

**75 ml/5 tbsp boiling water**

**1 large red, green, yellow or orange (bell) pepper**

**1 × 295 g/10 oz/medium can of carrots**

**A good pinch of dried mixed herbs**

**2.5 ml/½ tsp vegetable stock powder**

**A little water**

**Salt and freshly ground black pepper**

To serve:

**Wild rice mix**

---

1 Mix together the nuts, breadcrumbs, onion granules, soy sauce and oregano.

2 Blend together the spread, Marmite and 45 ml/3 tbsp of the boiling water. Stir into the nut mixture until it is thoroughly blended.

3 Halve the pepper and remove the stalk and seeds. Pack the nut mixture into the pepper halves. Put the remaining water in a small shallow dish and add the pepper. Cover with foil.

4 Bake in a preheated oven at 190°C/375°F/gas 5/fan oven 170°C for 30–40 minutes until the filling is golden-brown and the pepper is tender

5 Meanwhile, to make the gravy, purée the contents of the can of carrots with the mixed herbs and the stock powder in a blender or food processor. Tip into a saucepan and heat through, stirring. Thin with a little water, if necessary, to a pouring consistency. Season to taste.

6 Transfer the pepper halves to a plate, spoon the gravy around and serve with wild rice mix.

# Crushed Chick Pea Shishies with Fresh Mango Salsa

*A large can of chick peas makes enough for two people so, if you are eating alone, cook half and chill the remainder in a covered container for another day. The salsa will keep in the fridge for a couple of days too.*

---

### SERVES 2

---

For the shishies:

1 × 425 g/15 oz/large can of chick peas (garbanzos), drained

1.5 ml/¼ tsp onion granules

2.5 ml/½ tsp garlic granules

5 ml/1 tsp dried mint

5 ml/1 tsp dried oregano

2.5 ml/½ tsp ground cumin

30 ml/2 tbsp plain (all-purpose) flour

1 small egg white

Salt and freshly ground black pepper

About 60 ml/4 tbsp milk

25 g/1 oz/¼ cup dried breadcrumbs

A little sunflower oil for frying

For the salsa:

1 small fresh mango

2.5 ml/½ tsp onion granules

5 ml/1 tsp clear honey

5 ml/1 tsp Worcestershire sauce

15 ml/1 tbsp chopped fresh coriander (cilantro)

To serve:

Warm plain or sesame pitta breads, finely shredded lettuce, grated carrot and peeled, seeded and grated cucumber

1  To make the shishies, place all the ingredients except the milk and breadcrumbs in a food processor. Run the machine until a coarse paste is formed, stopping and scraping down the sides as necessary.

2  Shape the mixture into eight large oval sausage shapes. Roll each in the milk, then in the breadcrumbs to coat completely. Chill until ready to cook.

3  To make the salsa, cut the flesh off the mango stone (pit) in two or three pieces, following the shape of the stone. Score the flesh one way then the other into small squares, then bend back the skin and cut the flesh off the skin. Place in a bowl. If necessary, snip with scissors to cut up really small.

4  Add the onion granules, honey, Worcestershire sauce, coriander and a little salt and pepper. Mix well. Chill until ready to serve.

5  Heat just enough oil to cover the base of a non-stick frying pan. Fry the shishies for 6–8 minutes, turning once or twice, until golden. Drain on kitchen paper (paper towels).

6  Serve the shishies in pitta breads with shredded lettuce, grated carrot and cucumber and the salsa.

# Quorn-stuffed Aubergine

*This makes a delicious meal hot or cold so, if a whole aubergine is too much for you, enjoy the other half cold for lunch the following day.*

---

SERVES 1

---

*1 aubergine (eggplant)*

*10 ml/2 tsp olive oil*

*½ small sweet potato, grated*

*100 g/4 oz minced (ground) quorn*

*50 g/2 oz button mushrooms, sliced*

*2.5 ml/½ tsp onion granules*

*2.5 ml/½ tsp vegetable stock powder*

*75 ml/5 tbsp water*

*A good pinch of dried oregano*

*Salt and freshly ground black pepper*

*25 g/1 oz/¼ cup grated Edam cheese*

To serve:

*Feta Salad (see page 123)*

---

1 Put the whole aubergine in a pan of boiling water and cook for 4 minutes. Drain, rinse with cold water and drain again.

2 When cool enough to handle, halve lengthways and scoop out most of the flesh leaving a 'shell' with a thickish wall. Chop the flesh.

3 Heat the oil in a saucepan. Add the aubergine pulp, sweet potato, quorn and mushrooms and cook, stirring, for 2 minutes.

4 Add the onion granules, stock powder, water and oregano. Stir well and allow to bubble until the liquid has almost evaporated. Season to taste.

5 Put the aubergine shells in a shallow baking tin and pile the mixture in. Sprinkle the cheese over, cover with foil, taking care that the foil doesn't touch the cheese, and bake in a preheated oven at 190°C/ 375°F/gas 5/fan oven 170°C for 30 minutes until cooked through and the cheese has melted. Serve with Feta Salad.

# Marinated Quorn Steak with Chinese Vegetable Rice

*Quorn steaks always look very small but they are quite filling. For a large appetite, double the quantity of quorn and marinade.*

### SERVES 1

**10 ml/2 tsp sunflower oil**

**5 ml/1 tsp soy sauce, plus extra for sprinkling**

**2.5 ml/½ tsp clear honey**

**1.5 ml/¼ tsp ground ginger**

**1.5 ml/¼ tsp garlic granules**

**Freshly ground black pepper**

**1 quorn steak**

For the rice:

**50 g/2 oz/¼ cup long-grain rice**

**100 g/4 oz frozen Chinese stir-fry vegetables**

1 Blend the oil with the soy sauce, honey, ginger, garlic granules and a good grinding of pepper. Add the quorn steak, turn over to coat completely and leave to marinate for up to 1 hour.

2 Boil the rice in plenty of lightly salted water for 10 minutes, adding the vegetables half-way through cooking. Drain.

3 Place the quorn on foil on the grill (broiler) rack. Cook under a preheated grill for 2–3 minutes on each side, brushing with any remaining marinade, until cooked through and glazed.

4 Transfer the vegetable rice to a warm plate. Cut the quorn steak in diagonal slices and lay on top of the rice. Sprinkle with a few drops of soy sauce and serve.

# SIDE DISHES

All these dishes have been made to accompany the main course recipes in this book but, of course, they can be served with any plain grilled or poached fish, poultry or game birds to brighten them up enormously.

For salads, I have created dressings without vinegar, as it can often be a problem for IBS sufferers. If you can tolerate it then, please, use French dressing or vinaigrette if you prefer. Likewise, you may find you can tolerate mayonnaise – especially if it is a good-quality low-fat variety (like Hellman's Light). In which case, feel free to use it as an alternative to crème fraîche or yoghurt, or half and half, in the appropriate dressings.

# Rocket and Cucumber Salad with Italian Buttermilk Dressing

*If you find you cannot digest rocket as it is, chop it finely and mix it with the cucumber.*

| SERVES 1 |
| :---: |
| *15 ml/1 tbsp olive oil* |
| *15 ml/1 tbsp buttermilk* |
| *5 ml/1 tsp chopped fresh basil* |
| *A good pinch of garlic granules* |
| *Salt and freshly ground black pepper* |
| *5 cm/2 in piece of cucumber* |
| *A good handful of rocket* |

1 Whisk the oil with the buttermilk, basil and garlic granules. Season with salt and pepper to taste.

2 Peel and halve the cucumber, scoop out the seeds with a teaspoon and cut the flesh into small dice.

3 Mix together the rocket and cucumber and place on a small plate. Trickle the dressing over.

# Seeded Fine-shred Coleslaw

*You can make more of this and store it in the fridge for several days.*

SERVES 1–2

**5 ml/1 tsp sesame seeds**

**15 ml/1 tbsp sunflower oil**

**15 ml/1 tbsp low-fat crème fraîche**

**¼ small white cabbage, grated**

**1 carrot, grated**

**½ small green (bell) pepper, grated**

**1.5 ml/¼ tsp onion granules**

**A pinch of celery salt**

**Freshly ground black pepper**

1 Dry-fry the sesame seeds in a small pan until they turn golden-brown.

2 Tip into a bowl and stir in the oil and crème fraîche, then the vegetables and seasonings.

3 Toss the mixture thoroughly. Chill, ideally for 2–3 hours, before serving.

# Avocado Salad

*Cooling, refreshing and nutritious, this is a salad that goes with just about any main meal.*

| SERVES 1 |
|---|
| *1 small or ½ large avocado* |
| *2.5 cm/1 in piece of cucumber* |
| *A handful of watercress* |
| *15 ml/1 tbsp olive oil* |
| *15 ml/1 tbsp plain low-fat live bio yoghurt* |
| *1.5 ml/¼ tsp clear honey* |
| *A pinch of mustard powder* |
| *Salt and freshly ground black pepper* |

1  Halve and stone (pit) the avocado. Cut the flesh into dice.

2  Peel and halve the cucumber, scoop out the seeds with a teaspoon and cut the flesh into small dice. Chop the watercress.

3  Whisk together the remaining ingredients in a bowl. Add the prepared salad ingredients and toss gently.

# Feta Salad

*This is lovely with the Potato and Courgette Moussaka on page 76, or try it for a light supper with some warm pitta or daktalya (seeded Greek) bread. If you can eat tomatoes, do have some with this.*

---

SERVES 1

---

*1 wedge of iceberg lettuce, finely shredded*

*½ avocado, peeled and sliced*

*10 ml/2 tsp sliced black olives*

*50 g/2 oz/½ cup Feta cheese, diced*

*A pinch of dried oregano*

*15 ml/1 tbsp olive oil*

*Freshly ground black pepper*

1 Put the lettuce on a small plate. Scatter the avocado, olives and cheese over.

2 Sprinkle with the oregano, then trickle the oil over and add a good grinding of pepper.

# Braised Lettuce with Peas

*This is a French-style recipe. It is so good with plain grilled chicken, duck or fish.*

### SERVES 1

*1 small little gem lettuce*

*150 ml/¼ pt/⅔ cup chicken or vegetable stock, made with ½ stock cube*

*1 spring onion (scallion), trimmed and finely chopped*

*50 g/2 oz/½ cup frozen peas*

*1.5 ml/¼ tsp dried mint*

*Freshly ground black pepper*

1 Trim the stalk of the lettuce and cut the head into quarters.

2 Put the stock in a pan and bring to the boil. Add the lettuce and all the remaining ingredients. Bring back to the boil, reduce the heat, and simmer for 5 minutes.

3 Lift the lettuce and peas out of the pan with a draining spoon. Boil the liquid until well reduced and slightly thickened. Return the lettuce and peas to the pan, turn over in the sauce, then serve.

# Creamy Minted Mashed Peas

*Mashing peas before eating them is a good way of ensuring they don't cause you problems.*

SERVES 1

*50 g/2 oz/½ cup minted frozen peas*

*45 ml/3 tbsp water*

*30 ml/2 tbsp low-fat crème fraîche*

*Salt and freshly ground black pepper*

1   Put the peas and water in a small saucepan. Bring to the boil, reduce the heat and cook gently for 5 minutes, stirring occasionally. The water should have just evaporated.

2   Mash the peas with a fork and stir in the crème fraîche. Season to taste and reheat but do not boil.

# Warm Celeriac and Courgette Salad

*The rest of the celeriac will keep well in the fridge. It may brown slightly on the cut sides, but this can easily be trimmed off before use.*

SERVES 1

*15 ml/1 tbsp olive oil*

*¼ small celeriac (celery root), coarsely grated*

*1 courgette (zucchini), coarsely grated*

*30 ml/2 tbsp buttermilk*

*A good pinch of dried oregano*

*Salt and freshly ground black pepper*

1  Heat the oil in a small pan. Add the vegetables and toss over a gentle heat for 1 minute. Remove from the heat.

2  Add the buttermilk, oregano and seasoning to taste. Tip into a bowl and leave to cool for 5 minutes. Serve warm.

# Saucy Wilted Spinach

*Try this lovely side dish topped with a couple of poached eggs and served with a slice of toast for a light supper or lunch as well.*

SERVES 1

*100 g/4 oz fresh, well-washed baby leaf spinach*

*30 ml/2 tbsp crème fraîche*

*Salt and freshly ground black pepper*

*A little freshly grated nutmeg*

1 Put the spinach in a pan. Pour enough boiling water over to just cover. Bring back to the boil, then remove from the heat immediately.

2 Drain the spinach thoroughly in a colander, pressing the leaves well against the sides to remove excess moisture. They should still have a bit of shape and 'bite'.

3 Tip the spinach back into the pan and stir in the crème fraîche, a tiny sprinkling of salt, a good grinding of pepper and a sprinkling of grated nutmeg. Toss over a gentle heat and serve.

# Toasted Pepper Pasta

*Toasting peppers to remove their skins before cooking makes them much more digestible, so try this and enjoy it without, hopefully, any side effects at all. It is good served with some grated Mozzarella or fresh Parmesan shavings for a light meal too.*

SERVES 1

**1 small red (bell) pepper**

**1 small green pepper**

**15 ml/1 tbsp olive oil**

**1.5 ml/¼ tsp dried rosemary, crushed**

**Salt and freshly ground black pepper**

**75 g/3 oz pasta shapes**

**5 ml/1 tsp tomato purée (paste) (optional)**

1 Put the peppers under a hot grill (broiler) and grill (broil), turning occasionally, for about 15 minutes until blackened all over.

2 Pop them in a plastic bag and leave until cool enough to handle, then peel off the blackened skins. Cut the peppers into halves and remove the stalks and seeds. Chop the flesh.

3 Heat the oil in a small pan. Add the peppers, rosemary and a little salt and pepper. Cook gently, stirring, for 5 minutes.

4 Meanwhile, boil the pasta in lightly salted water according to packet directions until just tender but still with some 'bite'. Drain, then return to the pan.

5 Tip the peppers and their juices into the pasta with the tomato purée, if using, and toss. Serve hot.

# Black Mustard Noodles

*These are good with any Mediterranean or Middle Eastern main course. They have a lovely nutty flavour and the parsley adds colour and freshness.*

---

SERVES 1

---

*75 g/3 oz tagliatelle or other flat ribbon noodles*

*5 ml/1 tsp olive oil*

*5 ml/1 tsp black mustard seeds*

*A knob of reduced-fat olive or sunflower spread*

*Salt and freshly ground black pepper*

*15 ml/1 tbsp chopped fresh parsley*

1 Cook the pasta according to the packet directions. Drain in a colander.

2 Heat the oil in the pasta pan. Add the mustard seeds and fry until the seeds start to pop.

3 Tip the pasta back into the pan. Add the spread, a sprinkling of salt and pepper and the parsley and toss well over a gentle heat. Serve hot.

# Spinach and Raisin Sticky Rice

*This is delicious with the Chicken Satay on page 80 and is also good with the Soya Rissoles on page 110 and the Shishies on page 114. If you don't have any Thai rice, you can use ordinary pudding rice, though the flavour won't be quite as good.*

| SERVES 1 |
|---|
| *50 g/2 oz/¼ cup Thai Jasmine rice* |
| *175 ml/6 fl oz/³⁄₄ cup water* |
| *Salt and freshly ground pepper* |
| *100 g/4 oz frozen chopped spinach, thawed* |
| *15 ml/1 tbsp raisins* |
| *A pinch of grated nutmeg* |

1  Wash the rice well. Bring the water to the boil with a pinch of salt. Add the rice, stir and bring back to the boil. Part-cover and cook gently for 15 minutes, then remove the lid and cook rapidly for 1–2 minutes until the liquid has evaporated, stirring all the time.

2  Meanwhile, toss the spinach in a pan with the raisins for 3 minutes. Drain, if necessary, and return to the pan until the rice is ready. Tip the spinach mixture into the cooked rice, add the nutmeg and salt and pepper to taste and stir well. Heat through again, if necessary, and serve hot.

# Scalloped Potatoes with Herbs

*You could also cook this in the oven, in the traditional way, in a shallow baking dish or wrapped in a foil parcel at about 180°C/350°F/gas 4/fan oven 160°C – though a little higher would also be fine.*

### SERVES 1

*A small knob of reduced-fat olive or sunflower spread*

*1 potato, scrubbed and thinly sliced*

*1.5 ml/¼ tsp dried mixed herbs*

*Salt and freshly ground black pepper*

*75 ml/5 tbsp milk*

*15 ml/1 tbsp chopped fresh parsley*

1 Smear the spread over the base and sides of a small non-stick omelette pan.

2 Layer the potatoes slices evenly in the pan, sprinkling between each layer with the herbs and a little salt and pepper.

3 Pour the milk over and sprinkle with the parsley. Bring to the boil, turn the heat down as low as possible and cover with a lid or foil. Cook very gently for about 30 minutes or until the potato is really tender. Serve hot.

# Three Root Mash

*Ideally, reserve the vegetable cooking water for soup or stock as it is very nutritious and tasty. Try it topped with cheese or a poached egg for a light lunch or supper, too.*

### SERVES 1

*¼ small swede (rutabaga), peeled and diced*

*1 small parsnip, peeled and diced*

*1 turnip, peeled and diced*

*Salt and freshly ground black pepper*

*A knob of reduced-fat olive or sunflower spread*

*15 ml/1 tbsp low-fat crème fraîche*

1 Place all the vegetables in a pan, just-cover with water and add a pinch of salt. Bring to the boil and cook for about 15 minutes until really tender.

2 Drain thoroughly and return to the pan. Heat gently to drive off any last moisture, stirring all the time.

3 Mash thoroughly using a potato masher or fork, working in the spread.

4 Beat in a pinch of salt, a good grinding of pepper and the crème fraîche. Serve hot.

# Cabbage with Walnuts

*Cabbage will keep in the vegetable box in the bottom of the fridge for a good few days.*

SERVES 1

*1 small knob of reduced-fat olive or sunflower spread*

*5 ml/1 tsp sunflower oil*

*¼ small green cabbage, finely shredded*

*30 ml/2 tbsp boiling water*

*15 ml/1 tbsp chopped walnuts*

*Salt and freshly ground black pepper*

1  Heat the spread and oil in a small saucepan. Add the cabbage and toss over a high heat for 2 minutes.

2  Add the water and walnuts and cook quickly for 3 minutes, stirring frequently, until the liquid has evaporated and the cabbage is just tender.

3  Season to taste and serve piping hot.

# DESSERTS

You should try to avoid very rich, full-cream desserts and those with actual chocolate or coffee in them because they are likely to aggravate your symptoms. However, this does not mean that you cannot enjoy a delicious dessert after your main course.

Fruits are a good choice, especially when cooked or canned in natural juice, which shouldn't have the same effect as raw ones. Here you'll find a whole array of tempting – almost sinful – puddings to satisfy even the sweetest tooth.

# Apricot Almond Cooler

*This is like an elegant trifle but with no custard, cream or sponge in sight! You can try it with other soft dried or fresh fruits, such as sliced strawberries, raspberries or even nectarine or peach.*

---

SERVES 1

---

*4 ready-to-eat dried apricots, finely chopped*

*30 ml/2 tbsp white wine*

*2.5 ml/½ tsp clear honey*

*1 digestive biscuit (graham cracker), crushed*

*15 ml/1 tbsp ground almonds*

*A few drops of almond essence (extract)*

*A small carton of apricot low-fat live bio yoghurt*

*A little ground cinnamon*

*A tiny sprig of mint (optional)*

1 Reserve one piece of dried apricot for decoration and put the rest in a small bowl with the wine and honey. Mix well.

2 Put the crushed biscuit in a wine glass and mix with the ground almonds. Sprinkle with a few drops of almond essence.

3 Spoon the apricots and their juice over the almonds and biscuit so the mixture is thoroughly soaked.

4 Spoon the yoghurt on top and dust with the cinnamon. Pop the reserved piece of apricot on top and garnish with the sprig of mint, if liked. Chill until ready to serve.

# Light Creamy Honey Pots with Soft Fruit

*If you can't eat egg yolks, use just the white. You can omit the fruit, if you prefer, and just trickle the honey over the custard.*

---

SERVES 2

---

*90 ml/6 tbsp low-fat crème fraîche*

*90 ml/6 tbsp buttermilk*

*1 small egg*

*2.5 ml/½ tsp vanilla essence (extract)*

*20 ml/4 tsp clear honey*

*About 100 g/4 oz fresh soft fruit, sliced if necessary*

---

1 Whisk together the crème fraîche, buttermilk and egg with the vanilla and half the honey.

2 Pour into two ramekin dishes (custard cups).

3 Stand the ramekins in a frying pan. Pour enough boiling water into the pan to come half-way up the side of the pan. Bring back to the boil, then turn down the heat to low. Cover with a lid or foil and cook very gently for about 30 minutes or until just set.

4 Remove the ramekins from the pan and leave to cool, then chill.

5 When ready to serve, put a small pile of soft fruit on top of each and trickle a little honey over.

# Pear and Marzipan Parcels

*It's not worth making this for one; depending on how many peach halves are in the can, it's better to make five or six. The parcels can always be stored in the fridge for up to 3 days or frozen.*

MAKES 5–6

**1 × 410 g/14½ oz/large can of peach halves in natural juice, drained reserving the juice**

**100 g/4 oz/1 cup ground almonds**

**15 ml/1 tbsp thick honey**

**A few drops of almond essence (extract)**

**5–6 sheets of filo pastry (paste)**

**A little sunflower oil**

To serve:

**Low-fat crème fraîche or plain low-fat live bio yoghurt**

1  Dry the peach halves on kitchen paper (paper towels).

2  Mix the almonds with the honey, almond essence and 20 ml/4 tsp of the reserved pear juice to a thick mouldable paste. Shape the almond paste into rounds and place on each peach cavity.

3  Brush the sheets of filo with a little oil. Fold the sheets into halves and brush again. Wrap a peach half in each folded sheet, then transfer, flap-side down to a lightly oiled baking (cookie) sheet.

4  Brush with a little more oil and bake in a preheated oven at 190°C/375°F/gas 5/fan oven 170°C for about 15 minutes until crisp and golden. Serve warm with a dollop of crème fraîche or yoghurt and the reserved juice handed separately.

# Chocolate Sweet Soufflé Omelette

*If you can't eat egg yolks, just use the white; whisk it until stiff, then whisk in the honey and cocoa. You can turn it into a Black Forest Delight by spreading the omelette with a little reduced-sugar black cherry conserve before adding the crème fraîche.*

### SERVES 1

*1 large egg, separated*

*15 ml/1 tbsp clear honey*

*15 ml/1 tbsp cocoa (unsweetened chocolate) powder*

*A small knob of reduced-fat olive or sunflower spread*

*30 ml/2 tbsp low-fat crème fraîche*

1  Whisk the egg white until stiff. In a separate bowl, whisk the yolk with the honey and cocoa until smooth.

2  Using a metal spoon, fold the egg white into the yolk mixture until well blended.

3  Heat the spread in a small omelette pan. Add the egg mixture, spread it out gently and cook over a moderate heat for about 2–3 minutes until the base is set and golden, taking care not to let it burn.

4  Place the omelette under a preheated grill (broiler) and cook for about 2 minutes until risen and just set.

5  Slide the omelette out on to a plate. Quickly spread half with crème fraîche and fold over. Serve straight away.

# Peach and Almond Crumble

*It's not worth making this for one. If eating alone, you can have a portion every day for four days! It is also good with canned pears or apricots too.*

### SERVES 4

**1 × 410 g/14¹/₂ oz/large can of sliced peaches in natural juice, drained, reserving the juice**

**50 g/2 oz/¹/₂ cup flaked (shredded) almonds**

**25 g/1 oz/2 tbsp reduced-fat olive or sunflower spread**

**30 ml/2 tbsp clear honey**

**A few drops of natural almond essence (extract)**

**50 g/2 oz/¹/₂ cup ground almonds**

**50 g/2 oz/¹/₂ cup porridge oats**

To serve:

**Plain low-fat live bio yoghurt**

1 Put the peaches in a 1 litre/1³/₄ pt/4¹/₄ cup ovenproof dish. Sprinkle the flaked almonds over.

2 Mash the spread with the honey and almond essence. Work in the ground almonds and oats.

3 Spread the mixture over the peaches and bake in a preheated oven at 190°C/375°F/gas 5/fan oven 170°C for about 45 minutes until golden.

4 Serve with the reserved juice and plain yoghurt.

# Chocolate Mint Buttermilk Sorbet

*There is no point in making enough for only one portion. Simply keep the rest in the freezer until you fancy it to round off your meal on other days.*

---

SERVES 6

---

*30 ml/2 tbsp cocoa (unsweetened chocolate) powder*

*45 ml/3 tbsp boiling water*

*45 ml/3 tbsp clear honey*

*300 ml/½ pt/1¼ cups buttermilk*

*10 ml/2 tsp peppermint essence (extract)*

*2 egg whites*

---

1 Blend the cocoa with the water and honey. Stir in the buttermilk and peppermint essence.

2 Turn into a freezerproof container with a lid and freeze for 2–3 hours or until firm round the edges.

3 Whisk with a fork to break up the ice crystals.

4 Whisk the egg whites until stiff, then fold into the chocolate mixture. Return to the freezer and freeze until firm.

5 Serve in scoops in small glasses.

# Ginger Bread and Butter Pudding

*Again, this makes too much for one, so store the other one in the fridge for another day. It will keep for 3 days. You can cook it in a small ovenproof dish, if you prefer.*

---

**SERVES 2**

---

*2 slices of white bread*

*A little reduced-fat olive or sunflower spread*

*A handful of mixed dried fruit (fruit cake mix)*

*1 piece of stem ginger in syrup, drained and finely chopped*

*30 ml/2 tbsp of the syrup from the jar*

*1 egg*

*200 ml/7 fl oz/scant 1 cup milk*

*2 pinches of ground ginger*

---

1 Cut the crusts off the bread, if preferred (though it is not essential). Butter lightly with the spread, then cut each slice into four quarters.

2 Use two triangles to line each of two lightly greased ramekin dishes (custard cups).

3 Sprinkle the fruit and stem ginger over. Top with the remaining bread.

4 Whisk the ginger syrup with the egg and milk and pour over the bread. Dust each with a pinch of ground ginger.

5 Bake in the oven at 180°C/350°F/gas 4/fan oven 160°C for about 40 minutes until golden and set. Serve warm.

# Baked Pear and Chocolate Cream

*This is too much for one, so store the remainder in the fridge and enjoy it cold the next day.*

SERVES 2

**1 × 225 g/8 oz/small can of pears in natural juice, drained, reserving the juice**

**150 ml/¼ pt/⅔ cup low-fat crème fraîche**

**15 ml/1 tbsp cocoa (unsweetened chocolate) powder**

**10 ml/2 tsp clear honey**

**1 egg**

1 Put the pears in a small, shallow ovenproof dish.

2 Whisk the crème fraîche with the cocoa and honey, then whisk in the egg.

3 Pour over the pears and bake in the oven at 180°C/ 350°F/gas 4/fan oven 160°C for about 40 minutes or until set. Serve warm with the reserved juice.

# Mango and Banana Jelly

SERVES 2–3

*150 ml/¼ pt/⅔ cup water*

*15 ml/1 tbsp powdered gelatine*

*1 ripe mango*

*1 large banana*

*15 ml/1 tbsp clear honey*

*5 ml/1 tsp lemon juice (optional)*

1  Put 60 ml/4 tbsp of the water in a small bowl. Add the gelatine and leave to soften for 5 minutes, then either stand the bowl in a pan of gently simmering water and stir until the gelatine is completely dissolved or heat briefly in the microwave. Stir in the remaining water.

2  Peel the mango and cut all the flesh off the stone (pit). Put the flesh in a blender or food processor with the banana and honey. Blend until smooth.

3  Add the gelatine and water and blend again. Sharpen with a splash of lemon juice if you can tolerate it.

4  Pour into a container with a lid and chill until set. Serve spooned into glasses.

# Papaya with Soft Ginger Yoghurt Meringue

*This is fabulously different and doesn't take long to make. You can leave the papaya unprepared after removing the seeds and put a scoop of low-fat ice cream in the papaya cavity, before topping with the yoghurt meringue and glazing, if you like.*

| SERVES 2 |
| --- |
| **1 papaya (pawpaw)** |
| For the meringue: |
| **1 egg white** |
| **15 ml/1 tbsp ginger syrup from the jar** |
| **90 ml/6 tbsp plain low-fat live bio yoghurt** |
| **1 piece of stem ginger in syrup, drained and finely chopped** |

1 Halve the papaya and scoop out the seeds. Using a teaspoon, remove the flesh in pieces, leaving a 'shell'. Pile the flesh back into the shells and place the halves in small flameproof dishes.

2 Preheat the grill (broiler). Whisk the egg white until stiff. Whisk in the ginger syrup, then fold in the yoghurt and the chopped ginger.

3 Pile the yoghurt meringue over the papaya halves and grill (broil) for 3 minutes until golden and glazed on top. Serve straight away.

# BAKES AND SUNDRIES

Bread, cakes and biscuits are delicious
when home-made but many can be full
of fat and sugar. These, however, are
made using all the good things that
should help your condition, not
worsen it. What's more, baking is very
therapeutic so it's the ideal occupation
to relieve stress.

# Extra-good Oatcakes

*These are delicious any time of day – for breakfast, as a snack, or with cheese and fruit to round off a meal.*

**75 g/3 oz/³/₄ cup medium oatmeal, plus extra for dusting**

**15 ml/1 tbsp wheatgerm**

**A pinch of salt**

**1.5 ml/¹/₄ tsp bicarbonate of soda (baking soda)**

**15 g/¹/₂ oz/1 tbsp reduced-fat olive or sunflower spread, melted**

**60–75 ml/4–5 tbsp hand-hot water**

1 Mix together the oatmeal, wheatgerm, salt and bicarbonate of soda in a bowl.

2 Stir in the melted spread and the water to form a firm dough.

3 Dust the work surface with a little oatmeal and roll out the dough thinly. Cut into rounds using a 5 cm/2 in biscuit (cookie) cutter, re-kneading and rolling the dough as necessary.

4 Heat a non-stick frying pan. Cook a few at a time for about 3 minutes until firm. Carefully turn over (so as not to break them) and cook for a further 2–3 minutes.

5 Transfer to a wire rack and allow to cool. Store in an airtight container.

# Brown Oat Soda Bread with Poppy Seeds

*This lovely bread is best eaten the day it is made. The oatmeal gives added texture and is particularly good for IBS sufferers.*

---

MAKES 1 LOAF

---

*175 g/6 oz/1½ cups plain (all-purpose) flour, plus extra for dusting*

*175 g/6 oz/1½ cups wholemeal flour*

*100 g/4 oz/1 cup medium oatmeal*

*60 ml/4 tbsp poppy seeds*

*10 ml/2 tsp bicarbonate of soda (baking soda)*

*5 ml/1 tsp salt*

*5 ml/1 tsp clear honey*

*300 ml/½ pt/1¼ cups buttermilk*

*About 60 ml/4 tbsp milk*

*Oil for greasing*

1  Mix together the flours, oatmeal, 45 ml/3 tbsp of the poppy seeds, the bicarbonate of soda and the salt.

2  Gradually work in the honey and buttermilk to form a firm dough, adding enough of the milk to make a soft but not sticky dough.

3  Knead gently on a lightly floured surface. Shape into a 20 cm/8 in round and place on a lightly greased baking (cookie) sheet.

4  Brush with a little more milk. Make a cross-cut in the top of the dough and sprinkle with the remaining poppy seeds.

5  Bake in a preheated oven at 200°C/400°F/gas 6/fan oven 180°C for about 35 minutes until risen and golden and the base sounds hollow when tapped.

6  Transfer to a wire rack to cool a little. Serve warm.

# White Bread with Lots of Extras

*As I've said before, a mixture of white and wholegrains is good for most IBS sufferers. This one has the best of both worlds. Enjoy it toasted for breakfast or sliced thinly, with a scraping of olive or sunflower spread, for a teatime snack.*

MAKES 1 LARGE LOAF

*450 g/1 lb/4 cups strong white bread flour, plus extra for dusting*

*40 g/1½ oz/⅓ cup wheatgerm*

*7.5 ml/1½ tsp salt*

*5 ml/1 tsp easy-blend dried yeast*

*20 ml/4 tsp sunflower oil, plus extra for greasing*

*40 g/1½ oz/⅓ cup sunflower seeds*

*40 g/1½ oz/¼ cup currants*

*40 g/1½ oz/⅓ cup chopped mixed nuts*

*10 ml/2 tsp clear honey*

*350 ml/12 fl oz/1⅓ cups milk*

To serve:

*Reduced-fat olive or sunflower spread*

1 Mix the flour with the wheatgerm, salt and yeast in a bowl. Stir in the oil, seeds, currants and nuts.

2 Put the honey and milk in a saucepan and warm until it feels hand-hot.

3 Mix into the bowl with a knife to form a soft but not sticky dough, using your hands once the mixture starts to bind together.

4 Turn the dough out on to a lightly floured surface and knead well for 5 minutes until smooth and elastic.

5 Return the dough to the bowl, cover with oiled clingfilm (plastic wrap) and leave in a warm place for 1 hour or until doubled in size.

6 Re-knead, then shape into a loaf and place in an oiled 900 g/2 lb loaf tin (pan), cover loosely with oiled clingfilm again and leave in a warm place until the dough reaches the top of the tin.

7 Bake in a preheated oven at 220°C/425°F/gas 7/fan oven 200°C for about 30 minutes until risen, golden and the base sounds hollow when tipped out of the tin and tapped. Transfer to a wire rack and allow to cool.

8 Serve sliced and 'buttered'.

# Banana and Wheatgerm Muffins

*These are gorgeous for a snack or for breakfast and should help to make you feel good and satisfied.*

MAKES 12

*1 large banana*

*40 g/1½ oz/3 tbsp reduced-fat olive or sunflower spread*

*50 g/2 oz/½ cup sunflower seeds*

*75 g/3 oz/¼ cup thick honey*

*225 g/8 oz/2 cups self-raising wholemeal flour*

*5 ml/1 tsp baking powder*

*2.5 ml/½ tsp mixed (apple pie) spice*

*1 egg, beaten*

*About 45 ml/3 tbsp milk*

1 Mash the banana in a fairly large bowl. Add all the remaining ingredients and beat thoroughly with a wooden spoon or electric whisk until smooth.

2 Lightly grease non-stick muffin or deep tartlet tins, or line with muffin papers. Spoon the mixture into the tins (they should be nearly full). Bake in a preheated oven at 180°C/350°F/gas 4/fan oven 160°C for about 20–25 minutes or until risen and the centres spring back when lightly pressed. Transfer to a wire rack to allow to cool. Serve warm or cold.

# Almond and Raisin Oat Bites

*These will help keep you feeling in tip-top condition.*
*Although you will find them very moreish, you should find*
*only one square is enough for a snack as they are quite filling.*

---

MAKES 12

---

*100 g/4 oz/¹/₂ cup reduced-fat olive or sunflower spread*

*100 g/4 oz/¹/₃ cup thick honey*

*30 ml/2 tbsp clear honey*

*50 g/2 oz/¹/₃ cup raisins*

*50 g/2 oz/¹/₂ cup flaked (slivered) almonds*

*175 g/6 oz/1¹/₂ cups rolled oats*

---

1  Dampen an 18 cm/7 in square baking tin and line with non-stick baking parchment.

2  Melt the spread and both lots of honey together in a saucepan. Stir in the raisins, nuts and oats.

3  Press into the prepared tin. Bake in a preheated oven at 180°C/350°F/gas 4/fan oven 160°C for about 30 minutes until lightly golden. Mark into pieces, then leave to cool in the tin before cutting up. Store in an airtight container.

# Luxury Soft Florentine Cookies

*Although these are thin, they are packed with good things and are absolutely scrumptious. They don't have a chocolate coating, so shouldn't upset your tummy.*

| MAKES 12 |
|---|

**65 g/2½ oz/scant ⅓ cup reduced-fat olive or sunflower spread**

**45 ml/3 tbsp thick honey**

**15 g/½ oz/2 tbsp plain (all-purpose) flour**

**30 ml/2 tbsp low-fat crème fraîche**

**25 g/1 oz/3 tbsp raisins**

**25 g/1 oz/3 tbsp dried cranberries**

**25 g/1 oz/¼ cup shelled pistachio nuts, chopped**

**25 g/1 oz/¼ cup sunflower seeds**

**4 dried apricots, chopped**

1 Put the spread and honey in a saucepan. Heat gently, stirring, until melted, then bring to the boil.

2 Remove from the heat and stir in all the remaining ingredients

3 Line a baking (cookie) sheet with non-stick baking parchment. Put spoonfuls of the mixture well apart on the sheet and press down lightly with a wet palette knife.

4 Bake in a preheated oven at 180°C/350°F/gas 4/fan oven 160°C for about 20 minutes until golden brown. Leave to cool, then transfer to a wire rack.

5 Store in an airtight container.

# Sesame Seed Thins

*These lovely biscuits are low in fat and are delicious on their own or with fruit and/or yoghurt for dessert.*

MAKES 10

**45 ml/3 tbsp thick honey**

**25 g/1 oz/2 tbsp reduced-fat olive or sunflower spread**

**1 large egg white**

**15 g/½ oz/2 tbsp plain (all-purpose) flour**

**15 g/½ oz/2 tbsp wholemeal flour**

**15 g/½ oz/2 tbsp sesame seeds**

1  Melt together the honey and spread in a saucepan.

2  Whisk the egg white until stiff and gently fold in the melted mixture. Fold in the flours and seeds.

3  Line two baking (cookie) sheets with non-stick baking parchment. Put spoonfuls of the mixture well apart on the sheets. Spread out into rounds.

4  Bake in a preheated oven, one sheet above the other, at 190°C/375°F/gas 5/fan oven 170°C for about 15 minutes until golden round the edges, swapping the sheets over half-way through cooking, unless you are using a fan oven.

5  Leave to cool for 5 minutes, then transfer to a wire rack to cool completely. Store in an airtight container.

# Light Savoury Popcorn

*This is the best low-fat popcorn I know. Enjoy it as a snack any time of day. You may as well make a tubful and store it in an airtight container to eat over the next few days (if it lasts that long!). You can always make more in batches, but don't make too much in one go or it won't 'pop'.*

MAKES ONE TUBFUL

*1 good knob of reduced-fat olive or sunflower spread*

*25 g/1 oz/¹/₄ cup popping corn*

*1.5 ml/¹/₄ tsp celery salt*

1 Melt the spread in a heavy-based saucepan, swirling the pan so it spreads out.

2 Add the corn and celery salt. Put on the lid of the pan and cook over a moderate heat, shaking the pan occasionally, until the popping stops.

3 Tip into a large sealable container and leave to cool without putting on the lid. Once cold, seal the container.

# Pear and Apple Spread

*This is a good way to eat fruit that won't harm your system. It is also a delicious spread for anyone – IBS sufferer or not! It keeps for ages in the fridge. You can buy a very good version in health food shops, when you can't be bothered to make your own.*

MAKES 1 SMALL POT

*4 eating (dessert) apples, peeled, cored and chopped*

*4 ripe pears, peeled, cored and chopped*

*100 ml/3½ fl oz/scant ½ cup water*

*15 ml/1 tbsp black treacle (molasses)*

*10 ml/2 tsp powdered gelatine*

1  Put the fruits, 90 ml/6 tbsp of the water and the treacle in a small heavy-based pan. Bring to the boil, cover, reduce the heat and cook very gently for 20 minutes, stirring occasionally, until really pulpy.

2  Meanwhile, mix the gelatine with the remaining water and leave to soften.

3  Tip the softened gelatine into the fruit pulp and stir until completely dissolved.

4  Purée in a blender or food processor. Turn into a clean small sealable container. Leave until cold, then chill until set. Store in the fridge.

# Fresh Apple Relish

*A tiny bit of this with cheese or cold meat is delicious and not a drop of vinegar in sight! It will keep for ages in the fridge.*

MAKES 1 SMALL POT

*2 eating (dessert) apples, peeled, cored and chopped*

*1 cooking (tart) apple, peeled, cored and chopped*

*A good handful of raisins*

*2.5 ml/½ tsp onion granules*

*15 ml/1 tbsp thick honey*

*1.5 ml/¼ tsp ground ginger*

1 Put all the ingredients in a small heavy-based pan. Bring to the boil, stirring, then reduce the heat, cover and cook very gently for 10 minutes, stirring frequently.

2 Spoon into a clean sealable container. Cover, leave to cool, then store in the fridge.

# INDEX